10 YEARS YOUNGER

COSMETIC SURGERY BIBLE

JAN STANEK

WITH HAYLEY TREACY

Books

TRANSWORLD PUBLISHERS
61–63 Uxbridge Road, London W5 5SA
a division of The Random House Group Ltd
www.booksattransworld.co.uk

First published in Great Britain
in 2007 by Channel 4 Books
a division of Transworld Publishers

A CIP catalogue record for this book
is available from the British Library.

ISBN 9781905026326

Addresses for Random House Group Ltd companies outside the UK
can be found at: www.randomhouse.co.uk
The Random House Group Ltd Reg. No. 954009

The Random House Group Ltd makes every effort to ensure that the papers used in its books are made
from trees that have been legally sourced from well-managed and credibly certified forests. Our paper
procurement policy can be found at: www.randomhouse.co.uk/paper.htm

Printed and bound in Great Britain by
Clays Ltd, Bungay, Suffolk

2 4 6 8 10 9 7 5 3 1

The information in this book has been compiled by way of general guidance in relation to the specific
subjects addressed, but is not a substitute and not to be relied on for medical, healthcare, pharmaceutical
or other professional advice on specific circumstances and in specific locations. Please consult your GP
before changing, stopping or starting any medical treatment. So far as the author is aware the information
given is correct and up to date as at 1 January 2007. Practice, laws and regulations all change, and the
reader should obtain up to date professional advice on any such issues. The author and publishers disclaim,
as far as the law allows, any liability arising directly or indirectly from the use, or misuse, of the information
contained in this book.

CONTENTS

ABOUT THE AUTHOR

Mr Jan Stanek FRCS is an internationally renowned cosmetic surgeon who has been practising from his private clinic in Wimpole Street in London for more than twenty years.

Originally from the Czech Republic, Jan Stanek studied medicine at Oxford. It was while he was a student at Oxford that he became fascinated by the idea of combining the craft of surgery with the aesthetic expression of cosmetic enhancement and so decided to pursue the field as a specialist interest.

After qualifying as a doctor, Jan Stanek trained as a surgeon and spent the next nine years working in the National Health Service. He then became an assistant to a plastic surgeon in private practice, and worked in this capacity for several years, continuously learning and gaining wide experience in all areas of surgery.

In 1984, Jan Stanek set up his own clinic. To date he has operated on over 10,000 patients, and today his private practice, Surgical Aesthetics, operates entirely from GP referrals and personal recommendations.

In 1999, Jan Stanek became Visiting Professor in Aesthetic Plastic Surgery at Brno University in the Czech Republic. Here he has been involved in teaching a new generation of plastic surgeons about the art and craft of cosmetic surgery. From 2002, Jan Stanek chaired the department of Experimental Plastic Surgery at the University Faculty of Plastic and Reconstructive Surgery at Brno University.

Currently registered with the General Medical Council as a Specialist in General Surgery, Jan Stanek has lectured all over the world and has published many articles and books on cosmetic surgery. More recently he has become a familiar name to television audiences as the resident cosmetic surgeon on the hit Channel Four series *10 Years Younger*.

Jan Stanek currently lives in Oxfordshire with his wife and two daughters.

INTRODUCTION

The Channel 4 series *10 Years Younger* has brought the reality of cosmetic surgery to our television screens. It has demonstrated that for the right person, surgery is a successful way to improve appearance and increase self-esteem. I decided to take part in the series because I felt that it offered an opportunity to shine an honest light on what was involved in cosmetic surgery, and to address some of the common misconceptions about it. I believe that for the most part we have succeeded.

Those who take part in *10 Years Younger* undoubtedly experience an extraordinary change in their self-perception, as a result of what surgery, dentistry, hair, clothes and make-up can offer the right candidate. This book is written with that in mind: it should be used as a reference guide to help you understand surgery, but as one tool in a battery of anti-ageing techniques. First and foremost in this armoury are always a healthy diet, plenty of exercise and not smoking. This book picks up where diet and exercise can no longer help.

After all, cosmetic surgery is a field that is certainly not without its controversies and misconceptions. Perhaps the most common misconception about cosmetic surgery is that it will change your life. Let me put this straight: it won't. Cosmetic surgery can only improve the quality of life as a consequence of increased self-esteem and better interaction with other people, but this is, at best, indirect, and the two are not strongly connected. Any potential cosmetic surgery patient should equally be aware that surgery can also have the opposite effect, particularly if you have unrealistic expectations or you are unlucky enough to suffer from a post-operative complication, which can, in fact, make you become entirely unhappy with your appearance. This is the gamble you need to prepare for.

Another misconception is that cosmetic surgery can make you look like a famous personality. Put simply, the aim of cosmetic surgery is only to improve upon what is present. It should never be used to dramatically alter a person's appearance to look like someone else. I would advise that you avoid any surgeon who suggests otherwise to you. Cosmetic surgery is a delicate business of aesthetically improving your features, not a short cut to a new identity.

Some people also believe that cosmetic surgery isn't as safe as other forms of surgery. In fact, even though it is elective surgery for cosmetic benefit, it is, by definition, only as invasive as any other surgery and is subject to complications like any other. Nevertheless, most cosmetic surgeons try very hard indeed to prevent complications from occurring because they are aware that this type of surgery is rarely justifiable on medical grounds alone. They are also aware that results are subjective and dependent upon individual expectations, which are difficult to define and quantify. But you should be confident that with the right surgeon, cosmetic surgery is just as safe as (maybe even safer than) other surgery.

THE DIFFERENCE BETWEEN PLASTIC AND COSMETIC SURGERY

Two great plastic surgeons of the twentieth century, Sir Harold Gillies and D. Ralph Millard, defined the difference between reconstructive (plastic) surgery and cosmetic surgery as follows: 'Reconstructive surgery is an attempt to return to normal, [while] cosmetic surgery is an attempt to surpass the normal'. In other words, plastic surgery is concerned with reconstruction, and cosmetic surgery with improving aesthetics. Plastic surgeons try to restore function or return appearance to 'normal', or near normal, following an accident, illness or congenital malformation. Cosmetic surgery, on the other hand, is a form of psychological intervention. It is about improving upon the normal, in the first instance in the eyes of the patient themselves, and the main goal is to improve the patient's self-esteem. What many perceive as vanity is perhaps better understood from the medical viewpoint that such surgery can directly affect a patient's psyche, in the vast majority of cases enhancing the patient's quality of life as a consequence.

In the latter half of this book, we focus on what we call 'cosmetic procedures'. The distinction between cosmetic surgery and the cosmetic procedure is relatively straightforward. If surgery is defined as 'the manual treatment of injuries or disorders of the body, operative therapeutics, or surgical work', then it follows that any treatment that does less than this, i.e. is less invasive, is a cosmetic procedure. The Cosmetic Procedures section is where you will find information about what you can do to enhance your appearance if the thought of the operating theatre is a step too far.

THE HISTORY OF COSMETIC SURGERY

Surgeons have been improving facial aesthetics for thousands of years, but until the nineteenth century these improvements were nothing more than an unexpected by-product of plastic surgery conducted to improve function. We can credit the ancient Egyptians, working as far back as 3000 BC, with the first attempts to repair facial trauma, though these experiments were largely disastrous. From here, the history fast-forwards to India, where the Hindu physician and author Sushruta, working in c. 600 BC, detailed the efforts of physicians to reconstruct earlobes and noses that had been severed as a punishment dished out by the Hindu justice system of the time. Reconstructive surgery continued to develop and is recorded through Roman times, but the practice fell dramatically out of favour during the Middle Ages. A rebirth in research came with the Renaissance, with texts written in Turkish Islamic and Italian which show a deepening understanding of the treatment of gynaecomastia (the presence of breast tissue in males) and nose reconstruction.

Reconstructive surgery seems to have taken until the end of the eighteenth century to reach Europe, at which point its history began a slow but constantly evolving progress, as techniques became refined and environments improved. However, attempts at cosmetic improvement remained a secondary consideration (and therefore aesthetically disastrous) for many years to come.

Cosmetic surgery as a discipline in its own right doesn't begin to mature until the discovery of anaesthesia in the middle of the nineteenth century. Thereafter, cosmetic surgery expanded at a tremendous rate and operations became increasingly safe, as surgeons could concentrate on surgery knowing that patients were not in pain and that they were being looked after by anaesthetists. Procedures such as facelifting, eyelid surgery, rhinoplasty, abdominoplasty and ear surgery were in development from the turn of the twentieth century. During this time, progress was slow and the procedures were done largely out of sight, because of the general lack of acceptance of this type of intervention.

Before the Second World War, cosmetic surgery was considered unethical and even immoral. Nevertheless, some plastic surgeons practised it in secret, even though most of them denied being involved in it in any way. Many 'cosmetic surgeons' during this time had no form of medical training and so simply practised what they thought was right, often inventing new procedures by experimenting on their patients. However unsavoury, this period created the foundations for what we now know as cosmetic surgery.

With the Second World War came huge advances in surgical techniques. Surgery as a whole experienced a vast expansion mainly owing to the lessons learned from the treatment of war injuries, but also thanks to the introduction of penicillin and better anaesthetics. Gradually, surgeons applied their experience in trauma and major surgery to cosmetic surgery; however, their efforts remained hidden because of the entrenched media and public hostility to intervention. In the fifties, cosmetic surgery was the preserve of the rich and famous, who wanted the aesthetic benefits surgery could bring but wanted their use of it to remain a secret. And where Hollywood stars led, the public slowly began to follow.

By the sixties, technological innovations in cosmetic surgery had come to the attention of the media, and public opinion began to shift. One development to have a big impact was the introduction of the silicone breast implant in 1962, which meant that the dream of increasing breast size became a tangible reality. Another important development that significantly improved the aesthetic possibilities of the field was the discovery that the endoscope (a sort of small telescope with a camera attached) could be used in cosmetic surgery to create operations that left only small scars on the skin's surface. Perhaps the biggest impact on the public's perception, however, came with the possibilities presented by the introduction in the eighties of liposuction, which rocketed to being the most popular surgical procedure available today.

The history of cosmetic procedures arguably began with the manipulation of botulinum toxin after its discovery in 1895. The next major development was the introduction of injectable collagen, which was followed by numerous other fillers and countless other procedures. Recently, the ability to manipulate laser and heat energy has meant that cosmetic procedures are now more sophisticated than ever.

THE GROWING FIELD OF COSMETIC SURGERY

Cosmetic procedures and cosmetic surgery are now a regular feature of everyday life. But what are the reasons behind the rise in popularity we have seen in recent years? One is undoubtedly the fact that they tap into everyone's insecurity about their appearance. Another reason is the effect the media has had in demystifying the process and making cosmetic surgery more accessible than ever. The part that *10 Years Younger* has played in this is unmistakable. But it is also down to our shifting perception of what it means to be beautiful and what it means to grow old. For women in particular, looking good plays an important part in their psychological well-being. (In part this can explain the difference between the number of cosmetic procedures performed on women and men – the ratio currently stands at 20:1.) But even in society as a whole, there has never been a greater pressure on us to look young and look good. And, in a society where we have more disposable income than ever, where happiness is measured in part by success and where success is undoubtedly aided and signified by looking good, the demand for cosmetic surgery will inevitably rise. In fact, the demand has exploded.

There are many who do not understand why cosmetic surgery draws so much attention, and others who feel that it is immoral to interfere with nature for vanity's sake. Of course, these views are valid in some respects, and it is likely that opinion will remain divided for some time to come. But if current trends continue, it seems that a permanent positive attitude-shift towards cosmetic surgery is likely. In my opinion, this can only help the profession develop, refine and further improve its practice.

Having cosmetic surgery is a big step and should be considered carefully. This book is designed to help you understand what is involved, from initial consultation to post-operative appointment twelve months later. I hope that it will help you become a highly informed and discerning potential consumer. The better informed you are, the better your chances of avoiding the less professional practitioners in the field and, ultimately, the better the results of any surgery you have are likely to be. Therefore, I hope this guide furnishes you with most of the information you will need to consider as you come to your own informed and independent decision about whether cosmetic surgery is right for you.

Jan Stanek FRCS

London 2006

Author's note – You will notice that most of the statistics given in this book relate to cosmetic procedures performed in the United States. This is because, at the present time, there are no comparable figures for many specific procedures in Britain. Where appropriate, I have stated how many times a year I perform each procedure.

IS IT FOR ME?

It is important before you even phone a clinic or talk to a surgeon that you carefully consider your motivations for surgery and your expectations of what can be achieved, and preferably talk over your decision with both your family and your GP. I have put together a list of questions and other suggestions that you might find helpful during this process.

THINKING IT THROUGH

Q Do I really need cosmetic surgery?

A In a world where so much value is placed on looking good and feeling young, it is easy to believe that anyone could benefit from what a cosmetic surgeon can offer. But this is not the case. You must try to look at your appearance and objectively assess how bad the problem is. The central question is this: if you don't actually *need* to have anything done, then why should you? Factor in this thought, too: does it bother you all of the time, or is it just because someone mentioned it once? The latter is no reason to part with money and undergo surgery. If having thought about this you still feel the thing you are unhappy about has a psychological impact upon your emotional well-being, you probably have a good case.

Q Can other people see it?

A It might be worth considering whether other people can see the problem that you do. They are more likely to be able to offer an objective viewpoint, and so it might be worth canvasing the opinions of a trusted few. If they can see it, then in all likelihood so will a surgeon.

Q Do I have some other problem?

A Have you thought about whether it is an aspect of your appearance that you don't like, or whether you are, in fact, transferring your unhappiness from some other area in your life? For example, could it be that you actually feel depressed about work, or your relationship, but rather than confront this idea, you have transferred these feelings on to your appearance? If this is the case, you might well benefit from talking to a counsellor, psychologist or other medical professional about your feelings before considering cosmetic surgery any further.

Q Who am I doing this for?

A If you are considering surgery because someone else wants you to do it (either directly or indirectly), don't. This is your appearance you are thinking about altering, and you will have to look at it every day for the rest of your life. It should be no one else's decision but your own.

Q What effect will it have on my life?

A Cosmetic surgery will not change your life. It will not save your marriage, get you a new job, make you rich or prove that you are successful. If you are thinking about this because you want any of the above, cosmetic surgery is not right for you. If, however, you believe that altering something you have been unhappy with for some time might raise your self-esteem, then you have more of the motivations that a surgeon will look for when assessing your suitability.

Q Do I have the time?

A Although many cosmetic procedures can be done in a lunch hour, surgery is not the same. If you opt for it, you are going to have to take some time off from work to recover. You therefore need to think carefully about whether you can rearrange your work, family and social life, which will all be affected if you have surgery.

Q What do I expect cosmetic surgery will achieve?

A Cosmetic surgeons can only work with what you have. They cannot create miracles or turn you into someone else. You run the risk of being very disappointed indeed if you think that cosmetic surgery can radically change what you look like. It is important to be honest with yourself about what you hope surgery can achieve, and then work out if it is realistic by researching the possibilities of the procedure you are interested in.

Q Can I afford it?

A Cosmetic surgery can be an expensive business. Any reputable practice or clinic should be able to offer an up-to-date approximate price list, but bear in mind that prices quoted for a procedure normally do not take into account the extras, such as hospital and anaesthetist fees.

IN THE KNOW At your consultation, ask for an itemized bill that details what the extra costs are likely to be, so that you can take this away and work out at home whether you can afford it. While it is reasonable to expect to pay a set fee for a consultation, you should not feel pressurized to part with any more money at this point.

Q Am I prepared for the risks?

A Complications happen. Even if you are the best-prepared patient and have the best surgeon in the world, things can go wrong.

When you look through this book, take time to think about the risks. Imagine them happening, and consider how you would cope.

Q Am I prepared for the pain and recovery? Do I have the right support?

A Cosmetic surgery may be elective, but nevertheless it is real surgery. Before you look any better, you can expect to feel a lot worse. There could be pain, bruising, weeping, swelling and considerable discomfort on the road to recovery. Sensible patients follow to the letter the aftercare instructions given by their surgeon or practitioner, but you have to be prepared for what could feel like a long haul. For example, in the case of a deep phenol peel, this might mean bathing your red, raw face every few hours, or in the case of an abdominoplasty, lying in bed with drains oozing fluid coming from your stomach for a couple of days. The best results require committed aftercare, and you won't always be able to cope alone, so think about who can support you through the process before you decide to go ahead with it.

Q Am I physically fit and healthy enough to cope with this?

A Fit and healthy people recover quickly from surgery. Non-smokers recover quicker than smokers. Consider that your surgeon might ask you to get into shape or stop smoking just to have the surgery, and decide whether or not you are prepared to do that. I have lost count of the number of overweight women who come to me to ask for liposuction because they believe it is a shortcut to a slimmer figure. Liposuction is a serious procedure that you need to be healthy to cope with, so it is often inadvisable to perform surgery on someone who is very overweight and a smoker. A surgeon will certainly look more favourably upon someone who is already on the road to a permanently healthy body. If you want to make lasting improvements, make your surgery part of a wider plan to get fit and have a healthy future.

Ｑ Am I emotionally fit and healthy enough to cope with this?

Ａ You should consider the emotional rollercoaster you are likely to follow after your surgery. As many of the contributors to *10 Years Younger* will testify, after the initial excitement of having surgery there is a big dip in mood, which slowly improves with time as the results begin to show. Consider how you will cope with this, since it may well be at least a few weeks before you are able to look at yourself in the mirror and not see the signs of a recent operation.

Ｑ Is it worth it?

Ａ Finally, think about whether or not it is worth it. Weigh up the potential results against the potential risks – the physical, financial and emotional costs of surgery – and judge whether you still want to continue. If you do, it's probably time to talk your decision through with a few people.

TALKING IT OVER

Ｑ Who should I talk to?

Ａ Talk to people in your family who will need to know – any partner or potential carer should be first on the list. Ask them for their opinion, and factor their response into your considerations. Next, talk to your GP. They will be able to give you an objective view of what you want done, let you know if there is any local provision on the National Health Service, and possibly even refer you to a surgeon. Your GP might be involved in your long-term aftercare, so it is a good idea for them to know your plans anyway. Your GP might also advise that you talk to a counsellor or psychologist first. Don't be afraid of this – if your motivations are clear and you are a suitable candidate, it is unlikely that anyone will try to dissuade you.

Start researching the procedures you are considering, by reading the relevant pages in this and other books, searching the Web for information and reading magazines on the subject. You may also find it helpful to talk to some of the contacts and organizations listed on pages 322–5, such as the General Medical Council or the Healthcare Commission, and to ask potential clinics to send you information on the procedures.

When you have considered your motivation, decided what you would like to change and have an idea of how it can be done, and you have researched the surgeons, clinics and procedures you are interested in, then you can think about contacting a clinic or surgeon to talk about a consultation. If you do all this, you are on the road to a positive and successful cosmetic surgery experience.

COSMETIC SURGERY:
THE FACE AND HAIR

··

If you are considering cosmetic surgery, it's likely that the first area you will think about having work done is on your face. And now, more than ever, there are so many procedures and operations to choose from that it's vital you understand each one. In this section, therefore, you'll find the essentials of all the surgical procedures that are available to enhance your features. We start with a comprehensive look at the facelift and then examine each feature in turn, from your eyes and your nose down to your mouth and even your hair. At the end of each chapter, you'll find answers to some of the most frequently asked questions I hear in my clinic.

THE FACE

The effects of gravity alone can be cruel to the complexion, but combined with the face's daily work rate and constant exposure to the elements, it makes the challenge of staying young-looking an uphill battle, and one which is seldom advanced without a little help from the experts. The classic operation that many people opt for, which gets rid of the jowls and tightens the skin in the lower two thirds of the face, is the facelift, or _rhytidectomy_.

ABOUT YOUR FACE

Here's a scary thought as you light up that cigarette or drink that cup of coffee. Your face is the means by which you are identified in this world. It is what people visualize when they hear your name or refer to you in conversation; it travels in your passport, smiles in your driving licence, identifies you at work. It is also the main tool you use to communicate. But before you have even opened your mouth to talk, the skin on your face has spoken a thousand words. It can betray just how many holidays in the sun you've enjoyed, how many late nights you've had, even how often you don't bother removing your make-up at night. If you're unkind to your face, your sins will end up literally written all over your features. You keep your clothes washed, your car tidy, and your home clean in order to keep them in good condition and maximize the impression you make on others. Shouldn't you take the same care with your face?

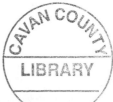

DID YOU KNOW?
Scientists have argued that faces can demonstrate six basic emotions: anger, fear, disgust, sadness, surprise and happiness. You may feel all of the above when you opt for cosmetic surgery!

HOW YOUR FACE AGES

- As you mature, your skin loses its elasticity and it also thins. This is because your skin doesn't produce as much natural collagen as it did in your youth.
- The underlying tissue weakens, forcing the tissues above them to clump, which causes wrinkles.
- Gravity begins to affect your face, pulling the skin downwards.
- The bone of your face becomes less dense, losing its volume, causing facial skin and soft tissues to begin to sag. This is how a saggy neck and jowls appear.
- Your body produces fewer melanocytes (pigment-forming cells), which can lead to uneven skin pigmentation, also known as 'age spots'.
- The blood supply to your face is reduced, resulting in a paler appearance.

Those old wives knew their stuff . . . sometimes. There is an element of truth in the tale that if you make a face for too long, or if the wind changes while you are doing so, it will stay in that position. The folds you create with your habitual expressions over time become ingrained in the outer layer of your skin, so that as you mature and your skin weakens, these folds leave permanent wrinkle reminders.

HOW TO GROW OLD DISGRACEFULLY

Here are some sure-fire ways to accelerate the ageing process:

Sun exposure This speeds up the natural ageing process, disorganizing the fibres in the deeper layers of the skin even more (a process called elastosis) and destroying dermal collagen. Sun exposure also leads to the outermost layer of the skin thickening unevenly.

Smoking Smoking reduces the amount of oxygen and vitamin C available in the blood, which will leave your skin a greyish-yellow colour and make it more likely to wrinkle.

Alcohol and caffeine Both of these dehydrate the skin, leaving it more susceptible to wrinkling. Alcohol and caffeine can also widen the blood vessels near the skin in the face, allowing unsightly thread veins to invade your complexion.

Stress and lack of sleep Stress will prevent you from getting the sleep you need for your body to repair and renew itself. This applies to the skin on your face, too!

Bad diet and lack of exercise A lack of vitamin C and iron will be reflected in a dull complexion. If you don't exercise, your circulation will be affected, which can also make you paler.

CONSIDERING SURGERY

There is a myriad of potential treatments for the face, from face masks to laser resurfacing. The only difficulty you are likely to come across is choosing between the many options on offer. When no amount of scrubbing, electricity or make-up will do, the most extreme option is, of course, the surgical facelift. But be warned: face lifting is not for the faint-hearted. Although fairly painless, the operation is uncomfortable for weeks after surgery and you will spend most of your recovery period looking like you've done a few rounds with a heavyweight champion. That said, hundreds of thousands of people opt for a facelift every year, and generally the results are deemed a big success in the great majority of patients.

DID YOU KNOW?
The skin on your face is twice as thick as the skin on your body.

THE EVOLUTION OF THE FACELIFT

The first facelifts were performed simply by excising skin from areas like the temples and in front of the ears and stitching the defect, thereby tightening the skin. This had a minimal effect, which was usually short-lived. After that, surgeons started lifting the skin as well and this produced slightly better results, though the problem remained that by stretching the skin only, the underlying soft tissues were still lax and so the skin appeared unnaturally tight. This is what became known as 'the wind-tunnel effect'. This skin-only facelift was first described in 1901 and, although refined, remained fundamentally the same until the seventies, when a new technique was introduced, the SMAS (superficial musculo-aponeurotic system) facelift. This procedure gave better results because it involved lifting some of the underlying tissue along with the skin of the face. Some problems remained, however, caused by tension on certain ligaments, especially in the cheek area, which produced an unnatural appearance of the cheeks.

Whereas standard facelifting really only improves the bottom two thirds of the face, recent advances in technique have incorporated deeper and more invasive work on all the features of the face. These newer techniques, particularly the endoscopic ones, demand more of the surgeon and are complex interventions. The post-operation swelling can be greater as a result, and in most cases it takes about six months before the final result becomes apparent.

DID YOU KNOW?
More than 150,000 Americans had a facelift in 2005.
Of those, more than half were between the ages of
51 and 64.

READY FOR LIFT-OFF . . . PREPARING FOR A FACELIFT

There are a number of things you can do before surgery that will benefit you as you recover from your facelift:

- If you smoke, now is a great time to stop completely. Smoking severely restricts the body's capacity to heal, and so the non-smoker is far more likely to recover quickly from the operation.

- Alcohol impairs your liver function, which makes you prone to bleeding, and caffeine quickens your pulse rate and raises blood pressure, so try to avoid either in the few weeks before surgery.

- Enlist a sympathetic partner/friend to help you through the surgery. Not only will they be able to physically help you immediately after surgery, but talking things through with someone will help your mental well-being considerably too.

- Establish a fitness regime a few months before surgery, so that you are in good physical shape before your operation. Stop as directed after surgery, before continuing in the months following your procedure. The fitter you are, the quicker you will recover.

- If you are overweight, try to attain a weight within the healthy range for your size before your operation. Not only is anaesthetic more risky if you are overweight, but losing weight prior to surgery will give you a better result from the facelift.

THE MODERN FACELIFT

In general the facelift operation refers to the tightening of facial skin and/or deeper tissues via incisions that run from the temples, around the ears, then behind and back into the hairline. However, it is fairly standard nowadays for a facelift to be combined with a neck lift, liposuction via a small incision under the chin, or other facial procedures such as a brow lift (page 64) or blepharoplasty (eyelid surgery, page 38), in order to enhance the entire face. Some surgeons call this a 'full' facelift. Other facelift procedures include the following:

Subcutaneous facelift First used over a hundred years ago, this is the oldest technique. The skin is cut in a line that runs from the temples, down in front of the ear, back round behind them and onto the scalp; the skin of the face is then lifted and tightened above and behind the ears, and the residual skin excised. This is an operation that is still used today, albeit rarely, in cases where more complex and invasive procedures cannot be justified because of health or age. In the right circumstances this operation can achieve a good result, but the results do not last as long as facelifts involving some kind of muscle tightening at the same time. It is more suited to older patients, or patients who have already had one facelift. One of the associated problems with this lift is that scars tend to stretch and become more visible, ultimately pulling the ears down.

SMAS facelift Introduced around thirty years ago, this is the modern standard facelift. It combines lifting the skin with tightening the underlying muscle and tissue (the SMAS). With this operation, the upper neck is also tightened and the skin draped over the entire lifted section. The advantage of the SMAS lift is that patients tend to look less 'stretched' and have less noticeable scars. This operation can also improve the appearance of the dreaded saggy neck a little, but it carries a greater risk of damage to the facial nerves than the subcutaneous lift.

Extended SMAS facelift (deep plane) This facelift was developed to address the issue of improving the cheeks and nose-to-mouth lines and creating a less stretched appearance. Here, the surgeon will lift the SMAS away from the cheek ligaments before tightening it up, thereby improving jowls, cheeks and nose-to-mouth lines. The operation is often combined with other procedures. With the right patient, it affords the best results in facelifting at present, scars are less obvious and recovery can be as quick as other forms of lift. However, the procedure is more invasive than the SMAS lift, and not all surgeons are able to do this operation.

Subperiosteal facelift Also known as the mask lift, this is a technique which attempts to lift the forehead and midface through incisions in the scalp and in the mouth. It works by moving the deepest layers of the face upwards together with the muscle and the skin. A scarless procedure, it is particularly useful in the younger patient with mid-facial problems. It produces the greatest change in appearance of the cheeks and is very effective on laughter lines, the eyes and nose-to-mouth lines. However, there is greater and longer-lasting swelling and a higher risk of nerve injury. The procedure also runs an increased risk of hair loss and permanent loss of sensation in the scalp, and it has little effect on jowls or a saggy neck. It is slowly being replaced by endoscopic and SMAS techniques.

Endoscopic facelift Recently, the subperiosteal lift has been refined in such a way that an endoscope, or small telescope with a camera, is fed through incisions in the scalp. Through another incision, the surgeon uses a long-handled instrument, which cuts beneath the lining of the bone (the periosteum) to avoid damaging the nerves and other structures. The surgeon works via a TV monitor. Smaller incisions have the advantage of smaller scars, of course, but there is still prolonged swelling with this operation. This is a procedure that not every surgeon will be able to carry out, and it is not yet known how long the results will last. Finally, with this operation, there have been reports of persistent numbness in the head and occasional temporary restriction of movement to some areas of the face.

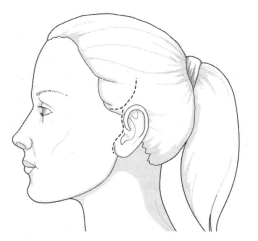

Incision locations for facelifts

THE RECOVERY PROCESS

It is best to try to sleep for the first few hours after the operation. The first twelve hours are the most critical recovery. You will stay in hospital overnight. The drains in your face will be removed the day after surgery. Before you go home from hospital, you will probably have your dressings removed and your hair washed. The surgery nurse will give you strict instructions on how to look after your facelift and it is imperative that you follow these to achieve a good result.

> DID YOU KNOW?
> The average facelift patient is in their fifties, but patients right up to their eighties and even nineties have been noted. Sometimes patients in their thirties have been treated, though this is rare.

Once you get home, you are advised to rest for the first forty-eight hours after the operation, preferably in a comfortable bed with your head propped up with pillows. You will need to sleep this way for a few days, since there will be extensive bruising, swelling, stiffness and numbness in the first few weeks after the operation, sometimes exacerbated by itching and headaches. Don't panic if you can't feel much at first: sensation should return to your face in a few weeks, or occasionally months, although this can vary from patient to patient according to the extent of the temporary nerve damage and the damage to the tissues of the face. Your stitches or staples will be removed after seven to ten days, and you will be able to return to work after two or three weeks.

RECOVERING FROM A FACELIFT: THE DOS and DON'TS
- **DO** make sure that someone can be at home to look after you immediately post-surgery.
- **DO** use extra pillows to prop up your head, and avoid turning in your sleep.
- **DO** drink plenty of water and eat a varied healthy diet to aid recovery.
- **DO** use an ice pack for short periods of time to reduce swelling.
- **DO** follow your surgeon's instructions on how to shower and/or bathe.

- **DO** try to keep your wounds clean through washing your hair as directed.
- **DO** take extra care when combing your hair to avoid the metal clips/sutures.
- **DO** limit your alcohol intake. It is best to avoid it altogether for a few weeks.
- **DO** take mild painkillers as suggested by your surgeon should you need them.
- **DO** contact your surgeon as soon as you notice anything untoward around the wounds such as pain, redness or a discharge.
- **DO** get plenty of sleep. You'll be giving your body time to repair and the best chance of a good recovery.
- **DON'T** talk or laugh – easier said than done, but the muscles in your face need a rest, too!
- **DON'T** do any kind of exercise for at least four weeks.
- **DON'T** allow your hair to get into the wounds behind your ears.
- **DON'T** use styling products on your hair for at least three weeks.
- **DON'T** dye your hair for at least six weeks.
- **DON'T** go out in the sun for at least two months. Use sunblock if you must go out.
- **DON'T** use any tobacco, nicotine patches or nicotine gum for a month.
- **DON'T** use aspirin or vitamin E supplements for three weeks.
- **DON'T** drive for at least two weeks.
- **DON'T** get on a plane for two weeks (so no retreating to the Med for convalescence!). You will need to be reasonably close to your surgeon in case you need to see him in the first few weeks after the operation.
- **DON'T** be tempted to get your teeth done at the same time. Avoid the dentist for at least six weeks.

A WARNING

A facelift cannot halt the sands of time for ever. Younger patients tend to see longer-lasting results, but ageing is a constant process that continues regardless of how many nips and tucks you opt for.

Many patients will find that they feel depressed in the first few days after a facelift operation. This is because their face still looks pretty battered, and the results are yet to be revealed. Most find that once the swelling eases, they are pleasantly surprised by the subtle effect a lift has had. However, occasionally patients are dissatisfied with the results of their facelift, believing that the surgeon has been too conservative. This is largely to do with the misconception that a facelift is a cure-all for every line and wrinkle, or that it can change a person's looks completely. A facelift will only rejuvenate what is already there, such as improving a haggard appearance through getting rid of jowls and a saggy neck. Trust in your surgeon – they are the best judge of how far to lift. After all, it really is in their best interest to make you look as good as possible without taking risks.

DON'T PANIC

The following are signs that you are recovering normally from a facelift:

- Swelling in the face
- Bruising in the face
- A sensation of tightness
- Yellowing skin behind the ears

Of course, if you feel any of these symptoms are more severe than they should be, contact your surgeon.

THE RISKS

Fortunately, there are few complications following a facelift, but some of the reported ones include the following:

- **Haematoma/bleeding** (See Glossary) This occurs in 1–10 per cent of cases.
- **Wound infection** It is rare (less than 0.2 per cent of patients) for a major infection to occur, but a localized infection is more common, especially behind the ears. This can easily be treated, with no long-term effects.
- **Pain** Sometimes patients experience persistent pain in the ears and cheeks.
- **Numbness** It is normal to experience some numbness to the face after the operation. Normally sensation will return when the nerves repair themselves.
- **Asymmetry** Some patients perceive asymmetry in their smile post-operation. This is often before the face has settled, but discuss it with your surgeon if it persists. Remember that everyone's face is asymmetrical both before and after surgery.
- **Poor scarring** Talk to your surgeon if you have found in the past that you heal badly. They will advise you of the potential scars after a facelift. Smokers are at greater risk of bad scarring.
- **Hair loss** Occurring near the temple scar, this is uncommon and usually temporary. Remember, however, that movement of the skin alters the hairline. This is often more problematic for men, who might find that they need to shave behind their ears.
- **Injury to the facial nerve** This complication can leave one of the muscles of the face paralysed temporarily or permanently. Discuss this complication with your surgeon.
- **Necrosis** (See Glossary)
- **Reaction to the anaesthetic** This complication is relevant to all surgery. Your pre-surgery consultation with your anaesthetist should lessen any likelihood of a reaction to the anaesthetic.

IN SHORT

The facelift operation is a popular, effective and highly refined operation that can dramatically improve your appearance. However, there is no gain without pain: not only is extensive aftercare required to achieve optimal results, but, prior to recovery, you will experience a prolonged period of discomfort. The operation itself is relatively painless and a number of advances in technique ensure that now more than ever a bespoke facelift can be created for every patient.

Generally facelift scars are good; however, they need to be looked after properly in order to avoid infection. Thankfully, there are few contraindications, though smokers are at a greater risk of complications and recovery will take longer. Among the risks associated with the surgery are swelling, numbness and, occasionally, injury to the facial nerve. So, as always, proceed with caution. Opt for surgery only when you have fully researched all of the suitable treatments, have been fully briefed and are completely happy to continue. That said, a facelift is a reliable solution for people concerned about their neck and jowls, and the results can completely transform the reflection you see when you look in the mirror.

FREQUENTLY ASKED QUESTIONS

Q How common is the operation?
A Facelifts are increasingly popular because results are more predictable than ever before and complications uncommon. This procedure is second only to blepharoplasty (eyelid surgery) for frequency of treatment in my clinic. I perform around two hundred of these operations a year.

Ⓠ How long does it take?

Ⓐ A facelift operation normally takes around three hours. More complicated facelifts can take up to six hours.

Ⓠ Is it painful?

Ⓐ Not really. The facelift operation is more uncomfortable than painful. Be prepared for the long haul, though: the settling-down process is a lengthy one and it will take you months to recover fully.

Ⓠ Will I have to stay in hospital?

Ⓐ In the large majority of cases, a general anaesthetic is used for this procedure, which means an overnight stay in hospital. Your head will be bandaged and there will be rather unsightly drains to be managed for the duration of your stay in hospital, so you'll probably be glad to be in someone else's care at first!

Ⓠ What can a facelift do?

Ⓐ A facelift will get rid of jowls and loose skin in the bottom two thirds of the face, restoring a more youthful look to your features and in particular your jawline. The facelift needs to be combined with other surgery in order to provide a full-face result. Some liposuction and/or a neck lift will improve neck rings and a 'gobble' neck. Only the more extensive facelifts can reduce nose-to-lip lines and improve the contour of your cheeks.

Ⓠ What can't a facelift do?

Ⓐ A facelift won't get rid of surface wrinkles. Nor will it rid you of sagging brows, or remove deep horizontal creases in the forehead or smoker's lip lines. A facelift will not remove excess fat around the eyes or wrinkles around the mouth.

Ⓠ Is there anyone who is not suitable for a facelift?

Ⓐ Patients who smoke have a higher risk of haematoma and necrosis of the skin (see Glossary). If you can't give up smoking completely, then the potential side effects can be limited if you stop smoking for one month before the facelift and one month after. Other conditions that your surgeon will want to know about include a history of Bell's palsy, hypertension or diabetes, all of which can have an effect on suitability. Finally, if you have been taking steroids for a number of years, then your surgeon might advise against a facelift.

Q What are the alternatives?

A If you feel faint at the sight of a scalpel, investigate the following to improve the skin on your face: the thread lift (page 275), chemical peels (page 231), botulinum toxin injections (page 299), dermal fillers (page 281), autologous cell therapy (page 290), ablative laser skin resurfacing (page 245) and fractional laser skin resurfacing (page 262).

THE EYES

As the ancient proverb says, the eyes are the windows to the soul. But if all anyone can see are droopy lids and bags as big as suitcases, people may be forgiven for thinking that that youthful glint and oozing charisma you used to have packed up and left long ago. The eyes are the first feature people notice about you – which is fantastic when you are in the first flush of youth, but not so great as you mature, when the constant work your eyes have done every day since you were born begins to be etched across your face.

ABOUT YOUR EYES

Our eyes are one of the organs we use to make sense of the world, and are therefore incredibly precious. Eyelids are like the eyes' personal protection service: their job is to shield and constantly wash the eyes, keeping them free of the dirt and grime in the atmosphere. The skin around your eyes is delicate, thin and stretchy. Eyes sit in a bone socket cushioned by fat, above the cheekbones. Around the eyes, a system of muscles and ligaments is hard at work pushing and pulling, steering your eyes to see and making you blink. And considering that we blink on average every six seconds, day in and day out, which equates to millions of times a year, this is one area of your face that is working pretty hard.

As we age, the elastic fibres that keep our skin taut become looser and tend to gather in formations. It is this gathering that creates the dreaded wrinkles and folds. The fatty cushion around the eyes can also slip to form bags under the eyes. If you combine this fragile skin with both the daily blinking effort and factors such as make-up application, contact lens wear, face washing, crying and exposure to pollutants, it's little wonder that the eyes are the first area on your face to start showing signs of wear and tear. And if you exacerbate the problem through smoking, which restricts the amount of oxygen in your blood, or sunbathing, which further weakens the fibres in your skin, you are actually accelerating the natural ageing process. So with all this daily abuse, are you really surprised you've got a few crow's feet when you look in the mirror?

FIVE WAYS TO HELP PRESERVE THE SKIN AROUND YOUR EYES

- Avoid squinting – it will only increase the skin's tendency to wrinkle. Wear sunglasses in bright conditions.

- Don't pull, rub or tug the skin around your eyes. Pat moisturizer on lightly.

- Always remove your make-up before going to bed.

- Avoid smoky or polluted atmospheres.

- Get more sleep.

TYPES OF BLEPHAROPLASTY

There are a number of treatments for the skin around your eyes. However, the surgical treatment available, called *blepharoplasty*, is a short and very common operation that can have a dramatic effect, with little pain and a brief recovery time. Blepharoplasty reshapes your eyes by removing redundant skin, fat and tissue around them. It is often performed on its own but can also be combined with other operations such as a facelift (page 23) or brow lift (page 64) to improve overall appearance.

DID YOU KNOW?
The term 'blepharoplasty' comes from the Greek *blepharon*, meaning 'eyelid', and *plastos*, meaning 'formed'.

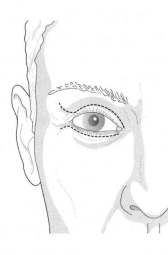

Blepharoplasty incision locations

There are many ways in which blepharoplasty can be performed. Each surgeon has their own likes and dislikes and they should be able to discuss these with you. In general, your surgeon will choose from the following types:

Upper eyelid blepharoplasty The surgeon makes an incision along the natural crease of the eye before removing a thin section of muscle, redundant skin and any excess fatty tissue. The wound is then closed with fine stitches.

Lower eyelid blepharoplasty An incision is made on the outside of the eyelid a few millimetres below the lash line. The eyelid skin is then lifted alone or together with the muscle beneath. Excess fat is removed. Finally, the skin is trimmed and reattached with stitches. Sometimes your surgeon may be able to stretch the skin around the eye slightly, which will improve the fine lines in the area, and reshape the eyelid more accurately. For this reason, the operation is generally more suited to older patients who have many problems that they wish to address.

Transconjunctival lower eyelid blepharoplasty The surgeon makes the incision on the inside of the eyelid. Excess fat is removed from under the eye, and the wound is closed with dissolvable stitches, or sometimes left to heal naturally. This method leaves no visible scarring, and the supporting structures of the lower eyelid remain intact. A technically more demanding operation, it is suitable for younger patients where skin and the underlying muscle are still quite elastic. If fine wrinkles are still present, these can be treated by ablative laser skin resurfacing (page 245) or chemical peeling (page 231).

Lower eyelid SOOF technique During this operation, which is normally used if the fatty pads underneath the eye have slipped downwards, the surgeon will move up these small fat pads, called the sub-orbicularis oculi fat, hence the title, thus reducing the eye's sunken appearance. This procedure is only used occasionally as a supplementary method to enhance the overall result and is considerably more invasive than routine blepharoplasty. It may be carried out either through the regular blepharoplasty incision or through the endoscopic approach, using an endoscope (a small telescope with a camera attached) to make two small incisions behind the hairline in the temple area.

Lower eyelid skin flap method The surgeon lifts away all of the eyelid skin, exposing the eyelid muscle. This allows the surgeon to manipulate or reduce the muscle and expose the fat pockets clearly before redraping the skin and removing the excess. This technique, which has an excellent safety record and results that are more than comparable to other techniques, is the method that I prefer to use.

THE RECOVERY PROCESS

No matter what type of eye surgery you opt for, the recovery time is similar. You will need to take a week or two off work while the bruising subsides. This will fade after ten to fourteen days. Most surgeons use non-dissolvable stitches and these have to be removed four to seven days after surgery. Sutures are removed early to prevent any permanent marking and allow the scar to be virtually imperceptible.

Once you are recovered, wave goodbye to those hereditary eye bags and say hello to a more awake-looking, brighter appearance. Your eyelids will probably feel less heavy, and if you had the lower eyelid blepharoplasty with an external incision, chances are you might have improved some of the wrinkling, too. But by far the best thing about this operation is that, because the scars are virtually undetectable, most people won't be able to tell that you have had something done. All they will notice is a more fresh and dazzling you!

FIVE TIPS TO AID RECOVERY

- A cold compress can be used to reduce swelling in the early stages of recovery.

- Bathing the area can ease discomfort.

- Eye drops can help (but check with the surgeon what type to use).

- You can take normal painkillers should you need to, as recommended by your surgeon.

- Stay out of the sun for at least three months after any type of surgery.

THE RISKS

Blepharoplasty is generally a very safe operation. As with any surgical procedure, there is a small risk of infection, but this is usually prevented by the use of antibiotic cream. Similarly, because surgery requires an incision, scarring is always a consideration. Fortunately, with blepharoplasty, the scars are virtually undetectable. It is very rare for blepharoplasty scars to become keloid or hypertrophic (red, angry, raised). Rarely, you might experience one or more of the following:

- **Dry eye** This is an occasional but not common occurrence immediately after blepharoplasty. It is usually temporary, and any prolonged dryness (which is rare) is easily treatable with artificial tears. Long-term contact lens wearers are more prone to dry eyes.
- **Drooping eyelid** Drooping can occur if too much skin is removed from the eyelid or the eyelid is weak. It usually corrects itself, but it might require taping during the early stages of recovery. Persistent drooping will need surgical correction.
- **Blurred vision** Patients occasionally experience temporary blurred vision.
- **Watery eye**s Sometimes fluid can collect beneath the membrane covering the front of the eye. It is usually caused by viral or bacterial infection of the conjunctiva. This can persist for a few weeks after surgery, but is easily treatable if persistent. However, most patients respond to steroid and antibiotic eye drops.
- **Numbness** At first you may feel some numbness around the site of the operation, but as the nerves repair themselves, normal sensation should return. It is very rare for the numbness to persist permanently.
- **Sunken eyes** If too much fat is removed from around the eye, the area can be left looking drawn.
- **Blindness** Another side effect that is extremely rare, but nevertheless has been reported, is blindness. Caused by bleeding behind the eyeball, it occurs in 0.0001 per cent of cases.

- **Reaction to the anaesthetic** This complication is relevant to all surgery. Your pre-surgery consultation with your anaesthetist should lessen any likelihood of a reaction to the anaesthetic.

> **DID YOU KNOW?**
> Arabic surgeons, working as early as the tenth century, first noticed that excess skin around the eyelids could affect vision, and they designed ways to remove it.

IN SHORT

Blepharoplasty is a routine, quick and relatively painless operation that is very common and popular. The reason for its popularity is the fact that the results are dramatic and there is minimal discomfort and little or no visible scarring. However, the procedure is not suitable for everyone, and there are risks, so, as always, proceed with caution. Opt for surgery only when you have fully researched all the other options, have been fully briefed and are completely happy to continue. That said, blepharoplasty is a good solution for people concerned about their ageing eyes, and the results really can roll back the years.

FREQUENTLY ASKED QUESTIONS

Q How long has the operation been around?

A Blepharoplasty was first described nearly two hundred years ago, as an operation to treat eye deformities. Over the years, the technique has been refined, first to treat the problem of overhanging eyelids and now for cosmetic purposes.

DID YOU KNOW?
The blepharoplasty operation can be adapted for people of Asian origin who desire a more Caucasian-looking eyelid.

Q How long does the operation take?

A You will be on the operating table for one to two hours for treatment to the upper and lower eyelids of both eyes.

Q How common is the operation?

A Blepharoplasty is probably the most popular procedure for facial surgery in the UK. I perform this type of operation around four hundred times a year.

Q Will I have to stay in hospital?

A Not normally. This operation is generally carried out under light anaesthesia or sedation with local anaesthetic, so most people leave the hospital the same day. The exact anaesthesia used depends on the surgeon's preference and the patient's fitness. If the procedure is to be performed in combination with other work such as a brow lift or facelift, a general anaesthetic is used in most cases.

Q Is it painful?

A Surprisingly, blepharoplasty is relatively pain-free. However, bruising and swelling can cause some discomfort in the early post-operative stages.

Q Is there anyone who is not suitable for blepharoplasty?

A If you suffer from glaucoma, have had problems with your eyes due to active thyroid disease or diabetes, or suffer from dry eyes or problem scarring, there is a higher risk of problems following the treatment. In that case, your surgeon might ask you to visit an ophthalmologist (a specialist eye surgeon) to assess your eyes for suitability for surgery.

Q What can't the op do?

A If sagging eyebrows or crow's feet are your problem, then blepharoplasty is not the answer. Sagging brows probably mean a brow lift would be better, and loose skin won't improve either. Similarly, if you suffer from dark circles under the eyes, your problem is probably not with skin and muscle; it may be caused by heavy pigmentation, transparent thin skin or visible fine blood vessels under the skin.

Q What are the alternatives?

A If you can't stand the thought of surgery, or are unsuitable for it, there are plenty of alternative weapons in the age-defying arsenal for the eyes. Non-surgical treatments include ablative laser skin resurfacing (page 245), botulinum toxin injections (page 299) and chemical peeling (page 231). You might even find that a few early nights and an increase in your daily intake of water do enough to improve the skin around your eyes without your having to resort to the laser or the scalpel.

THE NOSE

Squatting slap-bang in the middle of your face, your nose commands a lot of attention. It's your most prominent feature and is the second thing people notice about you, after your eyes. However, while the delicate area around your eyes responds well to a little TLC, your nose, made mostly of bone and cartilage, won't respond unless you force it. If you are the proud owner of a button nose, the good news is that it's your partner for life, but if it's an oversized nose that your family has passed on to you, you'll have to learn to love it, or opt for surgery if you want to do something about it.

> **DID YOU KNOW?**
> Doctors call the area from the corners of the mouth to the bridge of the nose the 'danger triangle' of the face, since it is possible for nasal infections to travel straight to the brain.

The good news is that noses age only a little. A few people find that as they get older, the tip of their nose begins to sink as the fat around the cartilage in the tip becomes absorbed, but this is rare. Opting for surgery that alters the shape of your nose, called *rhinoplasty*, is therefore not about making you look younger. This op is about either improving your nose function (also called *septoplasty*) or altering your nose to suit your face better (for cosmetic function). As such, it's an operation often performed on younger patients, and one with subjective results.

ABOUT YOUR NOSE

Your nose is a pyramid-shaped organ, with the upper third consisting of bone and the lower two thirds of cartilage. Your nose is used for breathing, in particular for warming the air that you breathe, and for your sense of smell. (When you smell something, air flows through your nose into the nasal cavity before it is turned into electrical impulses in the brain.) It is also the body's first line of defence from pollution, because, inside your nostrils, hairs catch airborne particles and prevent them from getting into the lungs.

The size of your nose doesn't normally affect its function, but the surgeon altering it must take extra care not to impair the organ. This is the reason why drastic changes to your nose shape are simply not advisable, and why results are usually only a compromise in this field.

FOUR REASONS WHY PATIENTS HAVE A NOSE JOB

- Hereditary problem: Some noses just run in families. There is little you can do yourself to improve your nose other than strategic application of make-up.

- Post-traumatic problem: This is caused by an injury to the nose. Some breakages can leave humps on the nose that can lead to an unsightly profile.

- Congenital problem: Repairing a nasal deformity such as cleft palate is another reason for nose surgery.

- Revision problem: This involves repairing an unfavourable result from a previous nose job.

ABOUT RHINOPLASTY

Although a fairly common procedure, the rhinoplasty operation is generally considered difficult, since access to the internal structures is restricted, function cannot be compromised and healing is unpredictable (to a small extent). Rhinoplasty ops can be performed by ENT (Ear, Nose and Throat) specialist surgeons and cosmetic surgeons alike, although ENT surgeons will be primarily interested in correcting functional problems rather than improving appearance. You are advised to find a surgeon who has performed plenty of rhinoplasties, as you'll want to be able to rely on the surgeon, while you are on the operating table, to judge how your nose would look best.

Rhinoplasty consists of the surgeon making small incisions in the nose, shaving off some bone and cartilage, and then breaking the bone and reshaping the cartilage to alter the nose shape. In most nose jobs, the surgeon will work on the tip of the nose first before working on the profile so that it fits in with the tip.

> **DID YOU KNOW?**
> The term rhinoplasty comes from the Greek *rhinos*, meaning 'nose', and *plastikos*, meaning 'to shape'.

TYPES OF RHINOPLASTY

Closed rhinoplasty Closed rhinoplasty means that no external incisions are made. Access to the inside of the nose is gained via incisions made inside the nostrils. From here, the skin of the nose is lifted from the cartilage and bone. The bone is chiselled and filed to shape, and fractured to achieve overall narrowing. If the septum (nose partition) is crooked, it can also be realigned via this operation. Tip cartilage is reshaped or removed, and the incisions are usually closed with absorbable stitches. The skin is taped and a splint is applied to prevent the nose from swelling too much. A small pack is sometimes inserted into the nose to prevent blood dripping. The major advantage of closed rhinoplasty is that there are no visible scars, so once the swelling has gone down no one will be able to tell that you have had surgery.

closed rhinoplasty   open rhinoplasty

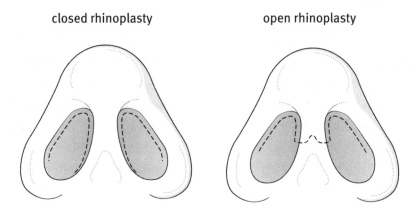

Incision locations for rhinoplasty

Open rhinoplasty With this operation, the surgeon makes an additional small cut across the columella (the skin between your nostrils that attaches your nasal tip to your upper lip), essentially joining up the two standard incisions on the inside of the nostrils. This allows the skin to be lifted away completely from the cartilage underneath. The advantage of this operation is that the surgeon can see more clearly, which is thought to allow more delicate alterations in the nose, especially in the region of the nasal tip, for example.

Tip surgery You may also hear your surgeon mention tip surgery, which is concerned solely with refining the tip of the nose.

Alar base reduction This is the removal of a wedge of tissue to narrow the nose at the base. It can be useful to balance out the width of the nose if you have had an excessively long nasal tip reduced, or to make very large nostrils smaller. The scars from this procedure should be hidden within the crease of your skin from the nose to the cheek.

THE RECOVERY PROCESS

When you come round from the operation, you will probably feel stiff, have packing in your nose to stem any bleeding and be sporting a cast to hold your new nose in place. It will be difficult to breathe through your nose, your face will be in the process of swelling up (it will be at its worst two days later) and two black eyes will greet your reflection in the mirror. The packing will probably be removed before you leave hospital.

TEN TIPS FOR GETTING OVER A NOSE JOB

In the first couple of weeks . . .

- Avoid bending or lifting as it will raise the blood pressure in your head.

- Try not to sneeze and try not to blow your nose.

- Avoid hot baths.

- Avoid hot food or drinks.

- Avoid alcohol, or at least drink only in moderation.

- Do not remove any crusting inside the nose until the cast is removed. Once the cast is removed, you can clean your nostrils with cotton buds as directed by your surgeon.

- Don't be tempted to have a peek under the plaster to see your new nose – it will look far worse in the early stages, and you could affect the result if you touch it now.

And in the long term . . .

- Spectacles can rest on the plaster cast while you have one, but after the cast is removed, tape them to your forehead instead of resting them on your nose for at least six weeks.

- Avoid body contact sports for at least three months.

- Use sunscreen on the tender skin on your nose until all the swelling has subsided.

When you get home, you are advised to rest in bed with your head propped up for a couple of days, and to apply a cold compress to ease the swelling and bruising as you need it. If you have pain, take paracetamol or distalgesics as directed by your surgeon. You'll be advised to avoid aspirin, or a painkiller containing aspirin, or any vitamin E supplements.

The cast will be removed after around seven to ten days. Any stitches usually dissolve, and the bruising will probably recede after around ten days, when you can return to work. Although the majority of the post-operative swelling will have gone after around three weeks, it will take at least six months for residual swelling to disappear.

It is important to remember that it is only possible to predict the outcome of rhinoplasty in general terms. Your surgeon may use computer imaging to indicate the look he is *aiming* for, but the nose you have a year after surgery largely depends upon how your nose reacts to the operation, and how well you heal. The results of this operation are permanent and so because of the vagaries of healing between 5% and 10% of patients find that they require touch-up surgery after a nose job. Unfortunately, revision can only be done a year after the original operation, as the scars need time to completely settle and the swelling to subside.

THE RISKS

Rhinoplasty surgery is very safe. Associated risks are uncommon and, for the most part, easily treatable. Some of them include:

- **Bleeding or oozing** Post-operative bleeding is usually stemmed by packing the nose.
- **Infection** Since the incisions are so small, infections are very uncommon and are usually cured by antibiotics. If synthetic grafts are used, there is a small possibility that these can become infected if they are rejected, which would mean revision surgery.
- **Scarring** Open rhinoplasties leave a tiny under-nose scar, which is virtually undetectable, and the scars from closed operations are hidden inside the nostrils. If you have thick skin that is prone to problem scars, you may be treated with steroid injections after the op.
- **Absorption or twisting of cartilage grafts** Sometimes grafts taken from the patient's body can be absorbed, which can lead to twisting in the nose. If the problem is bad, another operation may be necessary.
- **Difficulty in breathing through the nose** Some patients find that the difficulty in breathing through the nose that they experience in the immediate post-operative period can persist. It is more common when the nose has been narrowed or when scar tissue reduces the amount of air passing through the nostrils. This usually requires revision surgery.
- **Peeling nose** Sometimes, the skin of the nose can peel. Moisturizing the tender skin left will settle this peeling, which normally heals itself.
- **Pink nose** Sometimes tiny broken capillaries occur where the nasal skin is now thinner. This is easily corrected with laser treatment.
- **Numbness** Most patients can expect some temporary numbness following the operation.

- **Reaction to the anaesthetic** This complication is relevant to all surgery. Your pre-surgery consultation with your anaesthetist should lessen any likelihood of a reaction to the anaesthetic.

IN SHORT

Used to improve nasal aesthetic or medical function, rhinoplasty is a quick and painless operation that is extremely common and very popular. The results are reasonably subjective and so may involve revision surgery, but there is little or no visible scarring to contend with, and the associated risks are generally small and easily treatable. The procedure is suitable for virtually anyone who is unhappy with their nose, but reasonable expectations of what surgery can achieve are crucial. A rhinoplasty will not give you a new nose: it will only alter what you have, so, as always, proceed with caution. Opt for surgery only when you have a clear idea of how your nose can be improved and have researched whether what you want is achievable, and you have been fully briefed and are completely happy to continue. In general, rhinoplasty is a good alternative for people concerned about their nose, and the results have a dramatic effect on appearance in exchange for minimal discomfort.

FREQUENTLY ASKED QUESTIONS

Ⓠ How long has the operation been around?

Ⓐ Nasal surgery is one of the oldest surgical procedures. The first evidence comes from thirty centuries ago, in the form of a surgical papyrus from ancient Egypt referring to the diagnosis and treatment of nasal deformities. The history then moves from Egypt to India, where the physician and author Sushruta, working in around the sixth century BC, developed nasal-reconstruction procedures. The first surgeon to describe altering the size and shape of a nose to improve its aesthetics was Jacques Joseph at the turn of the twentieth century. Many of the basic rhinoplasty manoeuvres remain essentially the same today as when Joseph first described them. In the more recent history of rhinoplasty, in addition to regular refinements in techniques, debate has raged about whether open or closed procedures are better, with both falling into and out of favour at different times.

Q How common is the operation?

A Rhinoplasty is one of the more common cosmetic procedures, with over two hundred thousand operations taking place in the United States in 2005. However, it is also the operation with the largest revision rate: approximately one in ten rhinoplasties requires a return trip to the operating table for adjustments.

Q Will I have to stay in hospital?

A Some rhinoplasties take place under local anaesthetic and/or intravenous sedation, which avoids the need to stay in hospital overnight. However, many surgeons prefer to operate with a general anaesthetic, in which case you will stay in hospital to be monitored overnight.

Q How long does the operation take?

A Rhinoplasty is a time-consuming procedure, most often taking one or two hours to complete. More demanding rhinoplasty surgery can take up to four hours.

Q Is it painful?

A There is very little discomfort after a nose job. Most of the recovery is a quick but delicate process, but just because you feel fine after surgery, you shouldn't underestimate how delicate your new nose will be for the next six months.

Q What can rhinoplasty do?

A A cosmetic rhinoplasty can remove bumps or shorten, reduce, straighten, narrow, widen or enlarge the nose you have within limits.

Q What can't the op do?

A A rhinoplasty cannot give you the nose of your favourite soap or pop star. In altering the amount and shape of cartilage and bone in your nose, your surgeon can only work with what is already there. Drastic changes to the nose are both impossible and undesirable.

Q Is there anyone who is not suitable for rhinoplasty?

A Surgeons might be reluctant to operate on anyone particularly young or very old, or anyone prone to keloid (angry, red, raised) scarring. Although not normally a contraindication to surgery, thick skin can make a rhinoplasty procedure more difficult, since it tends to disguise the altered cartilage because it does not drape over the shape very well, and is more likely to form thick scar tissue during the healing phase. A greater consideration is the relatively high rate of revision surgery, so if you cannot face the possibility (or cost) of more than one trip to the operating table, think carefully before embarking on rhinoplasty.

Q What are the alternatives?

A If you can't bear the thought of paying to have someone break your nose, the only real alternative is to learn how the strategic application of make-up can improve your appearance – or learn to love your imperfection as the most interesting thing about you.

THE EARS

If there is one thing you can rely on children for, it's their honesty. So if you are the unfortunate bearer of a pair of very prominent ears, you can be sure they'll let you know about it. This is – possibly – funny if you are an adult who can laugh such comments off, but far from amusing if you are a child of school age and your ears cause you to be a victim of playground jibes. Consequently, *otoplasty*, the name used by surgeons for the operation to correct problem ears, is an operation often performed on children, although adult patients, many of whom have wanted the operation for many years, are increasing in number.

WHY EARS STICK OUT Prominent ears are caused by one of two things: either the patient hasn't got what is called the antithetical fold (the fold between the rim of the ear and the ear canal), or there is too much cartilage material in the concha (the inner concave part of the outer ear).

In surgical terms, otoplasty is a quick and relatively straightforward procedure executed for purely aesthetic reasons. It is not an operation that affects the function of the ear at all, because the part of the ear that we see has very little to do with hearing. Nor is it an operation that can make you look younger, since your ears don't really age you.

DID YOU KNOW?
Your ear normally measures around 5–6cm (2–2$^{1}/_{2}$ inches) in height, and protrudes at an angle of no more than 35 degrees from the head.

Otoplasty surgery for minors is generally conducted from the age of five. At this age, the ear has almost fully developed, and the underlying cartilage is still very supple and susceptible to manipulation. It is also a good age to consider surgery because it is usually only when children begin school that they become aware of their self-image. In adults, otoplasty is slightly more difficult, as the cartilage in their ears is stiffer, which makes it trickier to shape and reduces the blood supply to the skin and cartilage.

ABOUT YOUR EARS

The folded flap of skin with cartilage that sits on either side of your head is what most people refer to as the ear, though in reality this flap is useful only in directing sounds towards the inner ear. The ear can be divided into three parts, the outer, middle and inner ear. The visible flap we see, called the pinna or auricle, is part of the outer ear. It acts as a kind of funnel for directing sounds into the ear canal, through which sounds travel before being interpreted by the brain.

HOW AN OTOPLASTY IS PERFORMED

The surgeon will make an incision just behind the ear in the natural fold where the ear meets the head, and will then access the underlying cartilage. To achieve the desired affect, the surgeon can either remove or trim the cartilage if they perceive that the patient has too much, or shape and stitch back some of the cartilage to 'pin' the ears back along more natural contours permanently. Finally, the surgeon stitches up the initial incision and then places bandages on the ears.

DID YOU KNOW

If your problem is not with protruding ears but hanging ear lobes, surgical help is at hand. A cosmetic surgeon can easily cut away troubling excess lobe tissue, and stitch your lobe back together. It is usually done alongside another cosmetic procedure such as a facelift or rhinoplasty. Ask your surgeon about this at your first consultation.

BEFORE THE OPERATION Remember not to take any aspirin around the time of surgery – ears are prone to bleeding and aspirin will exacerbate this.

THE RECOVERY PROCESS

Since otoplasty is a routine operation, the recovery process is fairly quick and simple. When you get home, you should rest ideally for a couple of days sleeping with your head raised, to minimize the risk of bleeding. You will be asked to wear a head bandage for around seven to ten days, after which any non-dissolving stitches will be taken out. Your whole ear will probably feel tender and swollen for around a week, though normal paracetamol-based painkillers can be taken if you feel any pain, as directed by your surgeon. You may experience a tightening sensation as the day for your stitches to be removed approaches, but once they have been removed you will feel more comfortable. Most patients are back at work or school within two weeks. The ears will still be delicate for a few months, so avoid touching your ears and do not play any contact sports for a couple of months. Always contact your surgeon if you notice any signs of infection.

> **DID YOU KNOW?**
> After the operation your ears will move slightly as cartilage is so elastic and springy. It can take up to three months for ears to settle completely after surgery.

THE RISKS

- **Bleeding** Ears are particularly prone to bleeding, but this is usually localized and often resolves itself without intervention. Continued bleeding will have to be treated in the operating theatre.
- **Haematoma** (See Glossary)
- **Painful ears** Some patients experience persistent pain in their ears, particularly while the wound site is healing. If pain persists for a number of weeks, suddenly increases or cannot be controlled with painkillers, contact your surgeon, as it could be a sign of infection.
- **Unfavourable result** A common occurrence, this is mainly owing to a patient's expectations not being met by the result of surgery. Comprehensive and realistic pre-operative counselling will enable you to understand what can and can't be achieved.
- **Very asymmetrical ears** This can usually be corrected with a revision operation.
- **Skin problems** Sometimes skin on the ears can open and peel. This normally heals of its own accord.
- **Scars** There will be a thin white scar in the crease between the ear and the head. This is rarely a problem unless it grows to form noticeable lumps. You should talk to your surgeon before the

operation if you suffer from problem scars.

- **Infection** You are most likely to develop signs of infection three to five days after the operation. Symptoms include increased pain and swelling. Infection is rare and is usually treated through draining fluid and a course of antibiotics. Most surgeons use antibiotics after surgery as a preventative measure.
- **Numbness** It is possible that your ears may feel numb for a time after surgery, though this should soon pass.
- **Reaction to the anaesthetic** This complication is relevant to all surgery. Your pre-surgery consultation with your anaesthetist should lessen any likelihood of a reaction to the anaesthetic.

IN SHORT

The otoplasty operation is a quick and painless operation primarily used for children with prominent ears, though adults can also be treated. The results are generally good, but be aware that this operation will never make your ears perfectly symmetrical. There is little or no visible scarring, and the associated risks are small and easily treatable. The procedure is suitable for virtually anyone who is unhappy with his or her ears. However, as always, proceed with caution. Opt for surgery only when you have a clear idea of how your ears can be improved and have researched whether or not it is possible, and you have been fully briefed and are completely happy to continue. In general, the results have a dramatic effect on appearance for minimal pain or discomfort.

FREQUENTLY ASKED QUESTIONS

Q How long has the operation been around?

A The first cosmetic surgery for the ears was performed around a hundred and fifty years ago, and since then techniques have been constantly refined and altered to produce the efficient and quick operation we have today.

Q How common is the operation?

A The otoplasty operation is not particularly common, compared with other procedures such as facelift or rhinoplasty, though it is definitely increasing in popularity. I perform around ten otoplasties every year.

Q How long does the operation take?

A You should be in the operating theatre for one or two hours.

Q Will I have to stay in hospital?

A Otoplasty is generally carried out under local anaesthetic with sedation, so you'll probably return home the same day. For younger patients, the surgeon may recommend a general anaesthetic.

> **DID YOU KNOW?**
> Otoplasty surgery can be performed to create and/ or rebuild ears on patients who have no pinna (the visible flap), either through trauma or a congenital defect.

Q How long will the results last?

A Permanently.

Q What can otoplasty do?

A Cosmetic ear surgery can reshape the cartilage in ears with unnatural contours. It can also reduce large, stretched ear lobes or large creases and wrinkles in the ear.

Q What can't otoplasty do?

A Otoplasty cannot reduce the overall size of ears, nor can it make your ears perfectly symmetrical. Everyone has slightly asymmetrical ears anyway, so perfection is impossible.

Q Is there anyone who is not suitable for otoplasty?

A If you are in good general health, there is really no reason why you shouldn't undergo this procedure, although if you have any problems with your hearing, your surgeon will probably want to obtain a detailed history of the condition before deciding to proceed.

Q Is this operation available on the NHS?

A It is unlikely that as an adult you would be able to access this treatment on the National Health Service, but there is a greater possibility for children. In the first instance, contact your GP to discuss whether or not it might be possible on the NHS in your area.

Q What are the alternatives?

A There is a non-surgical treatment for prominent ears, but it is usually only possible just after birth. This is a Far Eastern practice of applying tape or bandages in early infancy to influence the growth and shape of the ear. The theory is that sustained restriction and pressure can guide the growth of the ear during infancy. However, there is no evidence that this approach is effective in most cases, and once ears have grown and cartilage has settled, this method is no longer an option anyway.

The late-nineteenth-century Dutch painter Vincent Van Gogh is famous for cutting off his own ear not long before he killed himself. His painting *Self-Portrait with Bandaged Ear* is not dissimilar to how you might look immediately after your operation!

THE BROW

If you have ever been asked why you look angry when you are not, or people tell you regularly that 'you look tired', then you might be surprised to learn that it is probably actually your brow, and not your mood, that needs a lift.

ABOUT YOUR BROW

The forehead is the third of your face where the effects of ageing are most noticeable. Unfortunately, it is also the area where there is very little that facial exercises alone can do to improve your appearance. We notice when jowls appear because they hang from the jawline, but your brow is far more deceptive. One day you barely notice it when you glance at your reflection as you walk out the door, and the next it's dropped and you are scaring passers-by.

DID YOU KNOW?
The average male forehead measures 7cm (2¾ inches) in height. The average height in women is 5cm (2 inches).

The reason is that when your brow droops it dramatically alters your appearance. It shortens your forehead, makes your face look square and sends your eyebrows retreating into your eye sockets. This leaves your upper eyelids heavy with flesh and increases the depth and number of wrinkles above your nose and between your eyes. If you want your forehead to return to its natural position and prevent the need to create eyebrows with make-up, the surgical solution you need to investigate is the brow lift. This is an operation that will lift your forehead and upper eyelids, reduce creases and frown lines, and weaken some of the muscles you use to frown, restricting your ability to create more unsightly lines.

HOW YOUR BROW AGES

Imagine that your eyebrows are teetering on a ridge of bone above your eyes. In your youth, the eyebrows happily stay in that position, since the muscles above them are strong and the skin is tight and resilient. But after around forty years, both the skin and the muscles in your face get tired and your features begin to succumb to the effects of gravity. Your brow can do little to fight this downward trajectory, and what results can be a dramatic and unsightly heavy ridge of skin and muscle above your eyes, or sometimes on your eyelids themselves. This will leave you looking tired and, worse still, constantly angry. And if you try to counteract this by lifting your eyebrows, you're putting yourself at a greater risk of developing unsightly horizontal lines on your forehead.

> **DID YOU KNOW?**
> When evaluating the face for cosmetic improvement, surgeons divide the face into three sections: the brow, the eyes and the lower face.

TYPES OF BROW LIFT

There are a number of approaches to brow lifting but, in general, surgeons consider one of two operations when deciding how best to make a brow lift work for you.

Coronal brow lift This is the traditional procedure. The incision is made in the form of an Alice band across the top of the head, usually behind the hairline, and the skin on the forehead is lifted. The skin is detached from the underlying bone, muscles that need to be removed are taken away, and the eyebrows are moved, before the excess skin is trimmed. The operation site is then closed with stitches or metal clips, and small drains are placed under the skin to drain off any excess blood. This technique allows the surgeon to manipulate or remove part of the muscles that can cause wrinkles, as well as lifting the eyebrows to a more natural level. Sometimes the surgeon will adapt the line of incision on the scalp to take account of the natural hairline and the amount of skin needing to be excised. This is an easy operation to combine with a facelift (see page 23): usually the surgeon joins incisions from the facelift above the ears. It is particularly suitable for those with high foreheads. However, the incision is long and the wound is large. Also, there is more extensive scarring, a higher risk of post-operative complications and hair loss, and an increased likelihood of scalp numbness. It usually requires an overnight stay.

Endoscopic brow lift This newer technique causes less trauma to the patient. Rather than one long incision, there will be around five or six, each about 2cm ($^3/_4$ inch) long, on the forehead, usually behind the hairline. An endoscope (a small telescope with a camera attached to it) is inserted into one of the incisions, giving the surgeon a clear view of the internal structures underneath. The procedure is done by observing a TV monitor with pictures relayed via the tiny endoscope camera. Using an instrument called a periosteal elevator, muscles and underlying tissues that are responsible for pulling the brow down are lifted and weakened. Then the bone lining under the eyebrows is released allowing the brow to rise. As such, there is very little movement of the skin, since the operation concentrates on the muscles underneath. The new position of the eyebrows is secured by either sutures or screws, inserted through one of the incisions within the hairline. (As part of the healing process, the forehead tissue that has been moved will attach itself to the bone in this elevated position, and so can produce a permanent lift.) Finally, the incisions are closed with stitches or clips. The smaller incisions mean less scarring than with the coronal brow lift, as well as less post-operative swelling. There is also reduced numbness, less likelihood of hair loss and a smaller risk of post-operative bleeding. Because of the shorter operating time, the endoscopic brow lift can be performed as a day case.

Some of the other procedures that your surgeon might consider include the following less popular options:

Browpexy This technique is used in conjunction with upper lid blepharoplasty (see page 38), sharing the incisions for the eye procedure to address the brows. The surgeon inserts several sutures in the brow in order to move the eyebrows to a higher position. Only a small elevation is possible, and so this procedure is particularly suitable for small asymmetries.

Brow suspension technique The surgeon secures the eyebrow in its new position via two small incisions placed in the flat part of the eyebrow. The sutures are then pulled through another incision, usually behind the hairline, and tied.

Corrugator resection This technique alters the amount of muscle between your eyebrows, thus preventing you from being able to frown and deepen present wrinkles. The incision is made in the upper eyelid crease or the hairline, or it can be done endoscopically.

Direct brow lift An incision is made just at the upper limit of eyebrow hair and an ellipse of skin is removed. When the wound is closed it causes the brows to lift. This procedure is not often used since the scar is potentially visible and other operations can offer better results.

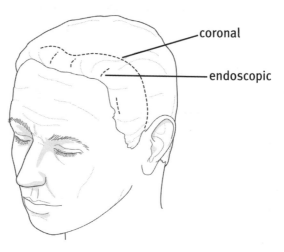

Incision locations for brow lift

THE RECOVERY PROCESS

You'll find that your head is lightly bandaged and a drain attached to your head when you wake up from the operation. Although you'll be able to leave hospital either on the day or the day after your surgery, it is possible that you will have to remove the dressings yourself one or two days later. After another couple of days, you'll be able to wash your hair and to shower. You will probably feel swollen and uncomfortable for this first week, and you can expect a tightening sensation around the stitches or clips as the day to have them removed approaches. This will ease once they are removed after around a week. There will be some bruising around your eyes, which will take around a fortnight to settle. You can expect numbness in your forehead, which should return to normal over the course of a few months. The amount of time it takes for recovery varies from person to person, but most patients will be able to return to work after around two weeks; this may be sooner if you have an endoscopic brow lift.

FIVE TIPS TO HELP YOU RECOVER FROM A BROW LIFT

- Keep your head upright, apply ice packs as needed and sleep with your head raised to reduce swelling.

- Use paracetamol-based painkillers, as directed by your surgeon, if you need them.

- Contact your surgeon if you notice any signs of infection or if you experience bleeding or bad pain.

- Ask, beg or pay someone to look you after for the first twenty-four hours you are at home after surgery.

- Avoid any exercise for at least three weeks after surgery.

THE RISKS

There are few risks following a brow lift, but some of the reported side effects include the following:

- **Hair loss** Occurring near incisions, this is uncommon and usually temporary, regrowing after around three months.

IN THE KNOW The best candidates for brow lift surgery are in their late thirties or early forties. At this age, the results will last longer.

- **Numbness** It is normal to experience some numbness of the face after the operation. Sensation should return when the nerves repair themselves.
- **Pain** A headache-like pain can be expected for several days after the operation. However, it is quite unusual to have pain afterwards and if it does occur, it can be controlled easily with painkillers.

- **Infection** It is rare for a major infection to occur (less than 0.2 per cent of patients). Localized infections, if they occur, can easily be treated, with no long-term effects.
- **Scarring** The scars following a brow lift are hidden in the hairline and so are not visible. However, if you heal badly, unsightly scars can occur. Patients who have the coronal brow lift should be aware that scars are potentially more visible with this procedure.
- **Asymmetry** Some patients perceive asymmetry in their brows after the operation. This is often before the face has settled, but discuss it with your surgeon if it persists.
- **Haematoma/bleeding** (See Glossary)
- **Necrosis** (See Glossary) Necrosis of the skin, which happens when the skin loses its supply of blood, has been reported, but it is very rare in brow lifting as the forehead receives an excellent blood supply.
- **Injury to the facial nerve** This is a complication that can leave one of the muscles of the forehead paralysed temporarily or permanently. You should discuss this complication with your surgeon.
- **Reaction to the anaesthetic** This complication is relevant to all surgery. Your pre-surgery consultation with your anaesthetist should lessen any likelihood of a reaction to the anaesthetic.

IN SHORT

The brow lift operation is a popular, effective and highly refined procedure that can dramatically improve your appearance. However, discuss with your surgeon the differences between the coronal and the endoscopic techniques and in particular your suitability for either. Both procedures have their advantages and disadvantages, though the fashion is moving towards the endoscopic technique as the scars are shorter and recovery time quicker. Sensible aftercare is required to achieve optimal results with this operation. Thankfully, there are few contraindications, though smokers are at a greater risk of complications and recovery will take longer. Among the risks associated with the surgery are bruising, hair loss and very occasionally injury to the facial nerve. So, as always, proceed with caution. Opt for surgery only when you have fully researched all of the suitable treatments, have been fully briefed and are completely happy to continue. In general the brow lift is a reliable solution for a drooping brow, and generally the results can make you look younger, less tired and, most significantly, a lot happier.

FREQUENTLY ASKED QUESTIONS

Q How long has the operation been around?

A A surgeon called Raymond Passot, working around the time of the end of the First World War, was the first person to describe the brow lift procedure and its benefits. His technique consisted of excising a strip of skin at the top of the forehead. This technique was refined through the years, mainly in conjunction with the latest thinking on facelifting. However, the advance that had the biggest impact was the introduction of the endoscope, which allows easy access to the operation site through small incisions and causes less trauma for the patient.

Q Will I have to stay in hospital?

A Most brow lifts are performed under a light general anaesthetic or a local anaesthetic and sedation. If your surgeon suggests a general anaesthetic, you may need to stay in hospital overnight for monitoring. Endoscopic brow lifting is carried out as a day procedure.

Q How long does it take?

A A brow lift operation takes one to two hours.

Q How common is the operation?

A More than 71,000 Americans had brow lift operations in the United States in 2005, making it one of the ten most common procedures. As yet there are no comparable figures for the UK, but I perform this operation around fifty to a hundred times a year, mostly endoscopically.

Q What can a brow lift do?

A A brow lift will make you look more awake and younger while eliminating that tired, angry or worried expression caused by a drooping brow. The operation will also help to reduce forehead furrows and raise the eyebrows. Sometimes the brow lift can address what you think is eyelid sagging, when actually it is caused by your heavy brow. In general, the procedure can change the overall proportions of the face, ultimately establishing a more attractive balance to your features.

Q What can't a brow lift do?

A A brow lift will not change the skin's surface, so it won't completely erase frown and furrow lines or get rid of scars or age spots. If this is where your problem lies, consider a chemical peel (page 231) or ablative laser skin resurfacing (page 245). Similarly, a brow lift cannot correct sagging eyelid skin; this condition requires the special attention offered by blepharoplasty (page 38).

Q How long will the results last?

A Although the brow lift has an immediate impact and a high satisfaction rate, your face will continue to age after your surgery, and although a brow lift can make you look younger than you did, it cannot stop the effects of ageing. The good news is that, if looked after properly, i.e. with no smoking or sunbed abuse, the rejuvenating results of a brow lift can last for five to ten years.

Q Is there anyone who is unsuitable for a brow lift?

A If you have had eyelid surgery before, your surgeon will want to assess how much skin can be lifted. Also, if you are a smoker, think carefully about whether or not to proceed. Patients who smoke have a higher risk of necrosis (see Glossary) and poor healing. Other conditions that your surgeon will want to know about include a history of Bell's palsy, hypertension or diabetes, all of which can have an effect on suitability.

Q What are the alternatives?

A If surgery is your last resort, there are a few options to try before you reach for the anaesthesia. Investigate botulinum toxin injections (page 299), currently the most popular treatment for forehead lines, and also look at dermal fillers (page 281).

THE CHIN

Many people who have real problems with their chin will probably have considered surgery long before the big Four-O. Chins fall into three camps. The first group consists of the lucky people who sport jaws in perfect proportion. Those in the second group have receding chins; for these people, implants and injectables may well address the problem. But if you are part of the third group, whose chins protrude in excess, it's surgery that you need to investigate.

ABOUT YOUR CHIN

Your chin gets its shape from the jawbone underneath the skin and the underlying muscle (mentalis). What shape you have is a question of genetics, but in general a male chin is slightly more prominent and square than a female chin. Aside from jowling, which is caused by the natural skin-slip we all have to contend with as the years go by, the chin doesn't really age, except for the quality of the skin. So the main objective of chin surgery is never to make you look younger; it's only to improve your profile and facial balance.

CONSIDERING SURGERY

If you are unhappy with your profile, chances are it's not just your chin that's causing you distress – you probably think your nose is pretty bad, too. This is because your nose and chin play an important part in facial balance. And if they're out of balance, there's probably some work that can be done on both. If your chin is weak, your nose may look big and if the nose is big the chin may look weak. In this case, though, you will probably head to a surgeon thinking only a nose job is required and may well leave the consultation planning for both a rhinoplasty and a chin implant.

Chin implants, alongside liposculpture (page 119) and cheek implants (page 83), fall into a category of surgery called facial contouring procedures. As they alter the dimensions and shape of your face, they are often performed in combination to enhance your profile. However, it is possible to perform any one of these procedures alone. Facial contouring is a delicate business if a subtle effect is to be achieved. Done well, the results can last a lifetime. Some implants have the added bonus of addressing deep folds and wrinkles and redefining areas of the face where volume has been lost with age.

However, there are cases in which liposculpture and implants cannot balance the face alone. In people with a particularly receding or protruding chin, a specific type of more extensive surgery is required. These operations can vary from a relatively straightforward chin reduction, where the surgeon reduces the size or position of the chin through manipulating the tip only, to far more extensive procedures which require the surgeon to slice through the bone of the chin in order to reset it back or forward. These procedures, called *chin advancement* or *osteotomy*, are carried out by maxillo-facial surgeons and are complicated procedures requiring lengthy recovery.

THE HISTORY OF CHIN IMPLANTS

Surgeons have been altering the contours of the chin since the thirties. At first the preferred implant was cartilage, but this was found to warp and twist quickly. Bone grafting was the next technique introduced; the grafts didn't warp, but they were gradually absorbed by the body. Surgeons were using prosthetics by the end of the forties, but these were often rejected by the body, eventually working their way out through the skin. In the sixties, surgeons began to use silicone implants. Silicone remains a popular implant today as it is easy to use and can be trimmed to fit. There are also currently a number of man-made implants available, which range from Gore-Tex to a substance derived from coral.

IN THE KNOW If you are having a nose job at the same time, your surgeon will operate on your chin first. This is so they can match the nose profile to the new chin, which is much easier than the other way round.

THE OPERATION

There are two approaches to chin implantation, depending upon where the surgeon accesses the chin from:

Intraoral approach Many surgeons prefer this method of implantation, for two reasons. First, the scar is on the inside of the mouth, so it reduces the chances of infection, which translates into a lower chance of complications occurring; second, it is easy to place accurately. The surgeon makes one incision no longer than 5cm (2 inches) on the inside of the mouth, between the teeth and the lower lip. A pocket is created beneath the bone lining (periosteum) of your chin to house the implant. The symmetry and position of the implant are checked, and the wound is closed with dissolvable stitches.

The submental route This approach is used where the operation is to be combined with another neck procedure, such as tightening the muscles in your neck or liposuction. It also allows for the implant to be placed in a lower position, if deemed necessary, and is some surgeons' preferred method of implanting. The chin is accessed from the bottom up, via an incision in the natural crease underneath the chin. The wound is closed with removable stitches.

IN THE KNOW... WHAT YOU CAN DO TO PREPARE FOR YOUR SURGERY There are a number of things you can do before surgery that will help your recovery. Think about trying the following:

- Stop smoking. You'll find it very difficult to smoke after the operation anyway, but if you have already stopped beforehand, not only will you have improved your body's ability to recover, you'll be on the road to a much healthier you.
- Enlist a sympathetic friend to help you through the surgery. Talking things through with someone will help your mental wellbeing considerably.
- Establish a fitness regime a few months before surgery so that you are in good physical shape for your operation. Stop as directed after surgery, before continuing in the months following your procedure. The fitter you are, the quicker you will recover.
- If you are overweight, try to attain a weight within the healthy range for your size before your operation, as having an anaesthetic is a more risky procedure if you are overweight.

THE RECOVERY PROCESS

If your surgeon operated via the submental route, you'll have a dressing strapped to your chin. But whichever approach was used, you will wake up from the operation with a swollen chin. Swelling is the body's natural reaction to the disturbance surgery causes. It'll be difficult to talk at first, and you'll need to stick to a soft-foods-only diet for around a week. You'll also probably be instructed to wear support tapes for a day or two after surgery, to hold the implant in place. You can expect to go back to work after a couple of days, though some people find they need a week to recover. If your surgeon used stitches under your chin, they will be removed after a week. Dissolvable stitches will dissolve in time. Residual swelling and numbness won't really settle for a couple of months, so the final result won't be apparent for some time.

> **DID YOU KNOW?**
> Surgeons might well use a study by a scientist called R. M. Ricketts in assessing your suitability for chin surgery. Ricketts said that if you draw a line from the tip of your nose to the tip of your chin, your upper lip should be just 4mm behind that line. The lower lip should be 2mm further back. How do you measure up?

After the operation, you should be vigilant with your dental hygiene, and make sure you finish the course of antibiotics your surgeon prescribes. Sleep with your head slightly raised to reduce any swelling, and wear your support tape for as long as instructed. Don't do anything that will raise blood pressure in your head, such as bending or lifting, for at least a fortnight. Take paracetamol or other prescribed painkillers if you have any pain. Avoid contact sports for a couple of months, and always contact your surgeon if you notice any signs of infection or you get a sudden increase in pain. Finally, avoid alcohol, or at least drink only in moderation.

THE RISKS

- **Infection** Although a general risk of all surgery, it is rare for an infection to occur. If the implant gets infected, it is difficult to treat the infection as it becomes a foreign body. In this case the implant has to be removed and the infection treated with antibiotics; the implant is then replaced after several months of healing.

- **Haematoma** (See Glossary)
- **Asymmetry** Some patients perceive asymmetry in their smile after the operation. This is often before the face has settled, but discuss it with your surgeon if it persists. It may be caused by the implant moving or twisting.
- **Numbness** Most patients find that their chin is numb after surgery. If the numbness persists, it could be a sign of nerve damage, though this is very rare.
- **Scar tissue tightening** Sometimes the scar tissue around the operation site can become tight, which in turn leads to the implant becoming distorted. However, this is a very rare complication. If it does happen, it may need revision surgery to correct.
- **Implant movement** A facial implant can sometimes move out of place of its own accord. Again, this may need revision surgery and the implant may have to be permanently fixed to the chin bone with a screw.
- **Scars** The scars from chin implants are either inside the mouth or barely noticeable short scars that sit right underneath the chin. They are easily camouflaged with make-up.
- **Reaction to the anaesthetic** This complication is relevant to all surgery. Your pre-surgery consultation with your anaesthetist should lessen any likelihood of a reaction to the anaesthetic.

IN SHORT

Chin augmentation is a simple and effective way of balancing an unsatisfactory profile. It is often used in combination with cheek implants and/or a rhinoplasty to correct various asymmetries in the face. Surgeons currently prefer man-made implants to cumbersome and unreliable grafting procedures, as synthetic implants are easier to manipulate and are less likely to be absorbed by the body. The operation itself can be performed as a day case, requiring either a small cut inside the mouth or an incision under the chin, which should eventually form a virtually undetectable scar. There are few contraindications to having chin implants. Among the risks associated with chin implants are swelling, numbness and occasionally implant shift. So, as always, proceed with caution. Opt for surgery only when you have fully researched all of the suitable treatments, have been fully briefed and are completely happy to continue. In general, chin implants provide a quick and straightforward solution for many people who are concerned about their chin and the effect it has on the overall facial balance. The results can positively transform your profile.

FREQUENTLY ASKED QUESTIONS

Q How long does the operation take?
A This surgery can take anything from thirty minutes to a couple of hours depending on the implant used.

Q Will I have to stay in hospital?
A Chin implants can be carried out under local anaesthetic with sedation, in which case you will be able to go home the same day. Even if you undergo the procedure with a general anaesthetic, you will probably be admitted as a day case.

Q Is it painful?
A Although sore in the immediate aftermath of the operation, if all goes well with the procedure implanting shouldn't cause you much pain or discomfort at all.

Q How long will it last?
A Chin implants are permanent if made of man-made material and so they should stay in a position that does not change with age.

Q How common is the operation?

A Although not extremely common, chin implants made it into the top twenty-five surgical procedures undergone by Americans in 2005, with more than thirty thousand operations performed. As yet, there are no comparable figures for the UK, but I perform this op at least twenty times a year.

Q What can a chin implant do?

A A chin implant will introduce volume into your chin, improving your facial balance, and making your nose seem less prominent. Sometimes it will also improve the appearance of wrinkles and dimples in the area and make your jaw look longer and the neck look more angled.

Q What can't a chin implant do?

A It will not improve the appearances of jowls, which are corrected through facelifting alone.

Q Is there anyone who is unsuitable for a chin implant?

A Chin augmentation is not recommended for anyone who has certain kinds of bone disorder. If this applies to you, talk to your surgeon to see if it affects your suitability. Also, if you are prone to problems with scars, your surgeon might recommend not having an operation. If you have a short jawbone and your bottom teeth are well behind the upper (doctors call this a malocclusion) it may be better to consider having your jaw lengthened by a maxillo-facial surgeon.

Q What are the alternatives?

A Dermal fillers (see page 281) can plump out the chin or cheeks to provide a balanced profile. Another alternative could be a direct fat transfer (page 108) into the chin from a donor site somewhere else in the body. More complicated procedures such as genioplasty or osteotomy can be considered if the chin severely recedes or protrudes.

THE CHEEKS

Your cheeks can betray your love of sunbeds, cigarettes or alcohol without your even saying a word. Unfortunately, the fleshy stretch of skin from your eyes to your jaw is also one of the first places on your face where your age begins to show. In youth, the skin is wrinkle-free, cheekbones are high and the flesh full, but with age the cheeks begin to droop and hollow out as the bone deteriorates. For some, the round cheeks Mother Nature provided are far from the ideal high cheekbones of models.

With age, the skin that sits just below the eyes on the cheekbones begins to give in to the effect of gravity and gradually slip. The face also begins to lose volume, the tissue underneath the skin gets weaker and the skin itself gets thinner.

> **DID YOU KNOW?**
> The medical term used to describe cheek augmentation is *malarplasty*. *Malarosteotomy* refers to the manipulation of cheekbones for a similar effect.

CONSIDERING SURGERY

There are a number of surgical options to redefine the contours of the cheeks. If cheek reduction is required, malarosteotomy procedures can manipulate the cheekbone itself, and liposuction can create a flatter cheek. If the cheeks need to be built up, malar or submalar implants are usually the first choice. More often than not, some degree of both building up and hollowing out is required. In this case, the surgeon will choose from any of these procedures in order to create a bespoke solution for your face. Cheek implants, alongside liposculpture (page 119) and chin implants (page 75), are part of a group of procedures for facial contouring. As they alter the dimensions of your face, albeit subtly, they are often performed in combination to enhance your profile or shape. However, it is possible to perform any of these procedures alone.

The purpose of cheek implanting is usually to make the cheekbones look either higher or fuller. Some implants can have the added bonus of addressing deep folds and wrinkles and redefining areas of the face where volume has been lost with age. Synthetic implants, particularly silicone, are the most popular implants in use today. Once inserted, they remain in the cheeks and do not get absorbed. However, be sure to discuss the advantages and disadvantages of the different types of implant with your surgeon, so you can be sure that you are getting the right implant for you.

Cheek implants can be placed in two positions on the face:

- **Malar implants** These are inserted in the outer upper cheek area to create the high-cheekbone look of many models.
- **Submalar implants** Inserted in the lower or mid-cheek region to help fill out a sunken face, these implants are often used to return a more youthful look to ageing features. Some surgeons prefer to use a fat transfer (page 108) to pad out the lower cheek area, believing that it creates a more natural look.

DID YOU KNOW?
Surgeons have been altering the contours of the face since the thirties (see page 10). Cheek implanting for cosmetic purposes was first reported in the seventies.

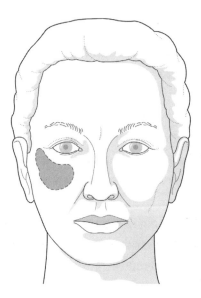

Location of cheek implants

THE OPERATION

The surgeon will access the cheek from one of four routes:

Intraoral approach This is the preferred method of inserting cheek implants. The scar is on the inside of the mouth and therefore undetectable. The surgeon makes an incision around 2cm (¾ inch) long on the inside of your mouth between the top teeth and the cheek. A pocket is created beneath the lining of the cheekbone to house the implant, the symmetry and position of the implant are checked and the wound is closed with dissolvable stitches.

CHUBBY CHEEKS If your problem is not so much very hollow cheeks as very chubby ones, there is a surgical procedure that could help. Some chubby cheeks are caused by the presence of a larger than normal fat pad called the buccal pad in the mid-face region. Surgeons are able to remove some of this fat pad during implant surgery, which will define the cheekbones more.

The extraoral route This is the procedure used when cheek implanting is combined with another surgery, such as blepharoplasty (see page 38). The cheek implant is inserted via the incision made on the outside of the lower eyelid. This operation allows for more accurate placing of the implants but also heightens the chances of complications. The wound is closed with removable stitches.

The preauricular approach Usually used in combination with a facelift, this procedure involves inserting the implants via the incision made for the facelift.

The transcoronal approach With this procedure the cheeks are accessed via the incision made for a brow lift (page 64) or a subperiosteal facelift (page 29).

THE RECOVERY PROCESS

You will wake up from the operation with a swollen face and numb upper lip. If you have tapes on your cheeks they will be removed after one to two days. Clean your mouth with a mouthwash for the first three days. After this, you can brush your teeth very gently, but try to avoid contact with your gums. It will be difficult to talk or laugh at first, and you'll need to stick to soft foods for around a week.

You can expect to go back to work after a couple of days, though some people find they need a week to recover. Dissolvable stitches will take some time to dissolve. Residual swelling and numbness won't really settle for a couple of months, but you should be able to appreciate the cheek enhancement soon after surgery.

TEN TIPS TO GET OVER YOUR IMPLANT OPERATION
- Be vigilant with your dental hygiene.
- Make sure you finish the course of antibiotics your surgeon prescribes.
- Sleep with your head slightly raised and apply ice packs as needed to reduce any swelling.
- Don't do anything that will raise the blood pressure in your head, such as bending or lifting, for at least a fortnight, and avoid contact sports for a couple of months.
- If you have any pain, take paracetamol or other painkillers your surgeon has prescribed.
- Take extra care not to burn your mouth when drinking hot fluids. Drink fluids with a straw.
- Avoid alcohol, or at least drink only in moderation.
- Limit talking and laughing.
- Avoid direct exposure to the sun for at least a couple of months.
- Contact your surgeon if you notice any signs of infection or you get a sudden increase in pain or swelling.

OPTIMIZING RECOVERY It is a good idea to visit your dentist before considering cheek implants to make sure your mouth is in good general health. Recovery will be quicker and easier if it is.

THE RISKS

The risks associated with cheek implants are the same as those following a chin implant (see pages 78–9), but there are no visible scars from cheek implants, since surgeons use the incisions from other operations or make the incisions on the inside of the mouth.

IN SHORT

Cheek implants are a simple and effective way of enhancing a flat cheek profile and are often used in combination with chin implants to correct various asymmetries in the face. Surgeons currently prefer man-made implants to cumbersome and unreliable grafting procedures, as synthetic implants are easier to manipulate and are less likely to be absorbed by the body. The operation itself can be performed as a day case, requiring either a small cut inside the mouth or an incision near the eye, which should eventually form a virtually undetectable scar. There are few contraindications to having cheek implants. Among the risks associated with implants are swelling, numbness and occasionally implant shift. So, as always, proceed with caution. Opt for surgery only when you have fully researched all of the suitable treatments, have been fully briefed and are completely happy to continue. That said, cheek implants provide a quick and straightforward solution for many people who are concerned about their cheeks, and the results can dramatically improve facial contour.

FREQUENTLY ASKED QUESTIONS

Q Will I have to stay in hospital?

A Cheek augmentation can take place under local anaesthetic with sedation, in which case you will be able to go home the same day. Even if you undergo the procedure with a general anaesthetic, you should also be able to go home the same day since the operation is not very extensive.

Ⓠ How long will I be in surgery?

Ⓐ Anything from forty-five minutes to a couple of hours, depending on the technique used and the surgeon.

Ⓠ Is it painful?

Ⓐ Although sore immediately after the operation, implanting shouldn't cause you much pain or discomfort, assuming all goes well with the procedure.

Ⓠ How long do implants last?

Ⓐ Synthetic cheek implants are permanent and will not deteriorate over time. However, the overlying soft tissues of your face will deteriorate and become thinner with age. In practical terms this means that your cheeks will become less prominent and more saggy with age.

Ⓠ What can a cheek implant do?

Ⓐ A cheek implant can make you look younger by introducing volume into your face, and will sometimes also improve the appearance of wrinkles and dimples in the area. In addition, having fuller and rounder cheeks is simply more attractive, especially in long faces with a flat cheekbone contour.

Ⓠ What can't a cheek implant do?

Ⓐ Cheek implants will not improve the surface of your skin, or get rid of crow's feet or nose-to-mouth lines.

Ⓠ Is there anyone who is not suitable for cheek implants?

Ⓐ If you are in good health and have realistic expectations of what implants can achieve, you are a good candidate for this procedure. Unfortunately, implants are not recommended for anyone who has certain bone disorders: talk to your surgeon to see if your suitability is affected. Also, if you are prone to problems with scars, your surgeon might also recommend not having the operation.

Ⓠ What are the alternatives?

Ⓐ Dermal fillers (page 281) can plump out the cheeks to provide a balanced profile. Another alternative could be a direct fat transfer (page 108) into the face from somewhere else in the body.

THE LIPS

Your lips are constantly drawing attention to themselves. They provide the frame for the picture your words describe, so if you're not happy with what nature gave you, lip enhancement could be one of the less invasive first treatments you consider as you investigate what cosmetic surgery can offer you.

Your lips are a sensory organ consisting of an upper strip and a lower thin strip of tissue used for eating and talking. More sensitive than anywhere else on your face, your lips require daily attention to look their best and prevent unsightly chapping. In youth, lips are full and voluminous, but as the skin gets thinner with age, the lips 'deflate'. If you accelerate the ageing process with smoking, you can expect to edge your deflating lips with lots of thin vertical wrinkles, the dreaded 'smoker's lines'.

CONSIDERING SURGERY

If you are seriously considering surgery for your lips, it's likely that you have already experimented with a temporary injection such as collagen or hyaluronic acid (page 284). If you haven't tried these temporary procedures first, they are definitely worth investigating before you book an appointment with a surgeon. It is also possible to have fat transferred from other areas of the body, usually the stomach or the buttocks, and injected into the lips. The fat causes temporary swelling, but it settles well, and because it is your own fat it isn't rejected by the body. However, this fat also tends to be absorbed after six to eight months. For more information on fat transfers see page 108.

For a more permanent effect, the choice is between an operation or a permanent implant. Operations are falling out of favour as the results are less reliable and the procedure is more cumbersome than implants, but they have been used to great effect in certain cases. Talk to your surgeon about both implants and surgical operations before you decide which is the best for you.

TYPES OF LIP OPERATION

Lip lift For people who have a long section of skin between their nose and lip line, a lip lift can offer good results. Surgeons remove a section of skin from just under the nose in order to curl the upper lip outwards, thus giving the illusion of a wider top lip, although the scar is problematic. This operation is used mainly for those who have a disproportionately long lip, sometimes following rhinoplasty (page 47).

Lip advancement The surgeon removes the skin just above or below the upper or lower lip border. When the wound heals there is a natural curling outwards of the lips, which can create a large pout. Since scarring is easily detectable with this operation, you would have to be prepared to outline the lips with liner every day if you had this procedure. The operation is best suited to those who have very thin lips with no cupid's bow, for whom a simple increase in volume will do nothing.

Lip reduction Suited to those with very large lips, this is essentially the opposite of lip advancement. If the lips are considered too fleshy, your surgeon can remove a strip of fat from the inside of the lip to pull the lips in.

ABOUT SURGICAL IMPLANTS

Surgical implants for the lips have been designed to take into account the fact that the skin of the lips is thinner than on the rest of the face, and also that the lips are always animated. Essentially the procedure for implanting material into the lips is the same. Your surgeon will make four tiny incisions at the corners of your mouth, before feeding the implant material through the lip, and then trimming the implant to fit and closing the wound. The choice of implant is likely to be from one of the following:

Autologous lip implant (autograft) This is an implant fashioned from the deeper layers of the patient's own skin, usually taken from the groin. This grafting procedure has the advantage that it won't be rejected by the body, but it does produce prolonged swelling and the deeper skin will probably thin with age, meaning that the effect it creates won't be permanent. Furthermore, it can leave you with a scar at the place from where the tissue was taken. This procedure has also been performed using muscle instead of skin. As with any surgical procedure, infection can occur, in which case the graft might not take, which would mean that the implant would need to be removed. This procedure is best suited to anyone who wants larger lips but does not want the temporary effect of injectables.

Donated human skin implant (allograft) There is a product available that uses donated human skin as an implant material. Pre-screened for viruses, this material is more likely to be accepted by the patient than a synthetic implant. These implants may have a tendency to become lumpy during healing, but this normally passes. As the tissue used is human, the body eventually absorbs some of it, and so the effect of the implant lasts for one to two years. This procedure is best suited to anyone who wants larger lips but does not want scars resulting from the removal of skin.

Synthetic implant The most common synthetic implant used for lips is a malleable form of Gore-Tex called expanded polytetrafluoroethylene, or ePTFE. Placed just under the lips, it is simply and easily implanted and the effect it offers is permanent, since this material will not be absorbed. However, that does increase the risk of its being rejected by the body, if infection sets in. Also, if placed awkwardly, these implants can move, sometimes working their way out of the skin altogether, although a synthetic implant can be removed if necessary at a later date. The procedure is best suited to anyone who wants larger lips but does not want to be implanted with human skin or to have scars resulting from the removal of skin.

Talk to your surgeon about which implant to go for. All surgeons have their own preferences, but don't be afraid to say frankly which one you would prefer.

THE RECOVERY PROCESS

Lip implants are a quick and simple procedure. When you go home, your lips will probably be numb and swollen, and since lip implants are stiff at first, you will find it difficult to speak, eat or drink. Try not to touch your lips or pick at them until they are completely healed. If non-dissolvable stitches are used, they will be removed after around a week. Do not hesitate to contact your surgeon if you notice any signs of infection.

THE RISKS

- **Movement** Sometimes a facial implant can move out of place of its own accord. This may need revision surgery to correct.
- **Scars** The scars where the implant incisions were made can be problematic since the skin in this area is sensitive and the lips are constantly moving. Though visible for several months,

these are tiny scars that should be barely noticeable and easily camouflaged with make-up.

- **Infection** Although a general risk of all surgery, an infection is rare and is easy to treat, with no long-term effects. Should an infection persist, the implant may have to be removed.
- **Reaction to the anaesthetic** This complication is relevant to all surgery. Your pre-surgery consultation with your anaesthetist should lessen any likelihood of a reaction to the anaesthetic.

> **DID YOU KNOW?**
> The skin on your lips does not have any sweat or sebaceous glands, which normally protect your skin. This is why your lips can dry out and become chapped so easily.

IN SHORT

Lip implants are a simple and effective way of plumping out thin lips. Surgeons currently prefer synthetic implants to lip operations, as synthetic implants are easier to manipulate and are less likely to cause problem scarring. The operation itself can be performed as a day case, requiring a few tiny incisions on the lip, which should eventually form a virtually undetectable scar. There are few contraindications to having lip implants. Among the risks associated with implants are swelling, numbness and occasionally implant shift. So, as always, proceed with caution. Opt for surgery only when you have fully researched all of the many alternative non-surgical treatments, have been fully briefed and are completely happy to continue. In general, lip implants can provide a quick and straightforward solution if you want to enhance your lips.

FREQUENTLY ASKED QUESTIONS

Q How common is the operation?

A Lip implanting is not a very common procedure, since injectable alternatives are relatively inexpensive and provide good results. I perform around twenty lip implant operations a year, mainly using the patient's own tissues.

Q Will I have to stay in hospital?

A You can have your implants fitted under local anaesthesia. You will not need to stay in hospital, and most people are back at work the next day, provided that the swelling is not too great.

Q How long does the operation take?

A You'll be in surgery for around thirty minutes to an hour.

Q Is it painful?

A Since a local anaesthetic is administered, you will not feel any pain during the procedure. In the days following surgery, however, your lips will be painful to touch. Any pain you feel after the surgery can be treated with painkillers as directed by your surgeon.

Q What can an implant do?

A The main benefit from this operation is an increase in lip volume, but the extra volume will also address some of the wrinkles around your lips.

Q What can't an implant do?

A Implants will not improve the contours of nose-to-mouth lines, nor will they improve the skin surface. Ablative laser skin resurfacing (page 245) is a better option for this. Lip implants cannot reshape lips that do not possess a natural cupid's bow.

Q Is there anyone who is unsuitable for lip implants?

A The lips can be a delicate area to treat, so proceed with caution if you suffer from problems with healing. Lip implants probably aren't the best idea if you suffer from active acne or recurrent cold sores. Similarly, if you have a dental problem, such as gum disease, it's probably best to treat this before you go ahead with a surgical procedure.

Q What are the alternatives?

A This is an occasion where surgery is secondary to the wide variety of non-surgical procedures for adding volume to the lips. Before you head for the operating table, consider a full-lip test-drive with a temporary injection such as bovine or human collagen or their alternatives. Many contributors to *10 Years Younger* have found that having veneers on their teeth has pushed the lips outwards, creating a more pleasing lip profile. If part of your problem is that you believe you have a sunken mouth, then perhaps a visit to the dentist before seeing the surgeon might be prudent. Finally, consider semi-permanent make-up. Edging the lips can create an illusion of fullness, which could provide the boost you seek without the need for injections or surgery at all.

THE HAIR

The effects of time alone can be cruel on the scalp, but if you combine this with the washing, drying, brushing and other grooming that your hair has to accommodate on a daily basis, it's unsurprising that virtually everyone will experience some kind of hair loss during their life. In response, a number of operations have been developed to treat baldness.

ABOUT YOUR SCALP

Your scalp is the section of skin that covers the top of your head, from the hairline at the front to the base of the neck at the back, and on the side to the top of your ears. This skin, which is well served with blood supply, is made up of five layers. The epidermis is the external layer. Underneath this, the dermis is composed of two layers. The first is a thin layer of fat and tissue. Under that, a thicker layer of more dense tissue connects the muscle at the front of your head to the back. The dermis is the layer of skin from which the hair on your head grows. Under here, another layer then separates this from the final, thin collection of fibrous tissue that covers your skull.

> **DID YOU KNOW?**
> Scalp surgery is also referred to as *galeoplasty.*

The scalp is not normally exposed to the elements, and so it doesn't really age in the traditional way, via wrinkling or sagging, since it is stretched very tight to begin with. Instead, it tends to show its age through shedding the hairs that normally cover it up.

WHY MEN GO BALD Men who go bald have hair follicles on their scalp that are sensitive to the male hormone dihydrotestosterone (DHT). This sensitivity is a genetic trait. When DHT begins to be produced by the body, those follicles that have a genetic predisposition to being sensitive can break down, which causes the hair itself to fall out. This can happen at any time after puberty.

ABOUT HAIR LOSS

For most women, hair quality tends to change when major hormonal changes take place in the body, such as menstruation, pregnancy, menopause or hormone replacement therapy (HRT). For men, patches of baldness usually occur in those with a genetic predisposition, handed down through the generations as a dominant gene. There are a number of treatments available for hair loss, both surgical and non-surgical. The current most fashionable treatment available, hair transplanting, can be used for both men and women whose hair is thinning or lost. But in the main, surgical procedures are used to treat *male pattern baldness* (MBP) or *androgenic alopecia*, which is the condition that leaves many men with a bald patch on the top of the head with hair at the sides and back.

WHAT CAN AND CAN'T BE ACHIEVED At your first consultation, aim to have a frank discussion about your expectations for treatment, to ascertain whether your surgeon believes that what you want is achievable. No technique currently available can grow new hair for your head. Essentially what all treatments do is make the little that is still on your head go a bit further. The best patients understand that surgery cannot give them the hair of their favourite film star; it can only provide extra coverage to an otherwise bald area. If your surgeon thinks you have unrealistic expectations, he may recommend not having the operation.

CONSIDERING SURGERY

Surgical treatments for hair loss are usually used in combination in order to provide a bespoke solution for each person. Broadly speaking, hair transplanting is performed on patients whose hair loss is not severe, and the more invasive surgical procedures are reserved for those whose baldness is more advanced. Currently surgical procedures for hair loss include hair transplantation, scalp flap surgery, scalp reduction surgery, scalp expansion and scalp extension.

DID YOU KNOW?
The following have all been used to promote hair growth, with little success: bird droppings, stinging nettles, human blood, bat's ears and even rat entrails.

HAIR TRANSPLANTATION

The most common procedure, this involves taking tiny grafts of the hair follicles on the head and then transplanting them into the areas of baldness. At one time, this technique left the patients with many little clumps of hair rather than a full head, but nowadays the grafts are so tiny and the surgeons so skilled that transplanted hair is virtually undetectable from natural hair, and there is minimum scarring. Because it is the follicle itself that is resistant to DHT, it doesn't matter where on the head a growing hair follicle is placed, it will continue to grow. However, the results of this procedure aren't always predictable and depend on a variety of external factors such as hair colour, texture and curliness.

The best candidates for hair transplanting do not have very advanced baldness and have areas of thick hair on their head. This makes this procedure a possibility for women who are experiencing thinning hair on their head. However, you are unlikely to be suitable if you have high blood pressure or blood-clotting problems, or you tend to suffer from bad scars. If you smoke, you are strongly advised to stop completely, or at least before and after your hair transplanting, as smoking restricts the flow of oxygen to the hair and could cause the grafts not to take.

THE OPERATION

Hair transplantation is normally carried out with a local anaesthetic and a sedative. First the surgeon will remove a good strip of hair-bearing scalp, usually at the back of the head where the hairs are quite thick. This strip can be many centimetres long, but is no more than a couple of centimetres (about ¾ inch) wide. The wound is closed with stitches. Grafts are then created by slicing the strip into sections, sometimes as small as one or two hairs thick. Finally, the grafts are inserted via tiny incisions into the bald part of the scalp. Because the operation involves literally inserting a couple of hairs at a time, you can expect to be in surgery for many hours.

THE RECOVERY PROCESS

You won't feel any pain during the transplant, but you can expect both the donor site and the transplanted areas to be pretty sore when the local anaesthetic wears off. You'll be able to go home as soon as the operation is over, though you'll probably have to wear a bandage on your head for the first day. It's a good idea to have someone with you on the day of your surgery in case you need any extra support and to drive you home. Most people find that they are able to go back to work the next day, though some people take a couple of days off if the scalp swells a lot. In these first few days, if your surgeon says that it is all right, take paracetamol-based painkillers if you have a headache, and apply any antibiotic ointment given to you. Do not shampoo your scalp until around three days after your operation and do not hesitate to contact your surgeon if your scalp is especially painful or you think there is an infection.

THE RISKS

- **Grafts don't take** Sometimes isolated follicles, or small patches of follicles, die, in which case the baldness returns. In this case, surgery needs to be repeated.
- **Hair loss** Normally the transplanted hair will fall out before new hair grows in its place.
- **Scars** Sometimes small bumps form at the transplant sites. These are usually camouflaged by the hair itself eventually.
- **Swelling** Because the scalp tissue has been manipulated, it is entirely normal for some swelling to occur. Some people find that their eyes become puffy for a few days, too.
- **Scabs** Sometimes scabs form over the transplant site. Although unsightly, they should crust and fall off of their own accord.
- **Infection** The scalp can become infected after a procedure, though this is rare. It would normally be treated with antibiotic ointment or oral antibiotics.
- **Reaction to the anaesthetic** This complication is relevant to all surgery. Your pre-surgery consultation with your anaesthetist should lessen any likelihood of a reaction to the anaesthetic.

> **DID YOU KNOW?**
> Hair transplants have been taking place since the thirties. At that time, however, the grafting was done to replace eyebrows and eyelashes in patients who had severe scarring after trauma.

SCALP FLAP SURGERY

This is a procedure used mainly for men who have receding hairlines. The surgeon will free a section of hair-bearing scalp that has plenty of healthy hair on it and reattach it at the front, while preserving its blood supply. A dramatic approach with immediate results, this is serious surgery and not for the faint-hearted. The approach is most often used in the treatment of traumatic hair loss (for example, to treat scars caused by burning) or hereditary hair loss defects. It works best when combined with hair transplanting or with scalp extensions or expansions. At one time, scalp flap surgery was used only to treat traumatic hair loss, but nowadays it has been used in patients with male pattern baldness or receding hairlines. It is not normally an option for female hair loss.

THE OPERATION

The classic operation is called the Juri flap and is normally performed in three stages over three weeks. The surgeon takes a long, narrow strip of hair from the back of the head, turns it around and reattaches it at the site of the new hairline at the front of the head. There are, however, alternative techniques that are done in two stages and are equally successful. Scalp flap surgery is usually performed under general anaesthesia, requiring an overnight stay in hospital.

THE RECOVERY PROCESS

A scalp flap operation is uncomfortable. When you wake up from the operation, you will have a large bandage strapped to your head. For the next couple of days, you will need to wear a hat, and you can expect headache, bruising and swelling. As the scabs form around the wound sites, your head will probably itch. You will not be able to wash or comb your hair for at least a week, and you will probably be advised to avoid contact sports for around a fortnight. You should follow the course of antibiotics the surgeon will prescribe and use painkillers, again as directed by your surgeon, should you feel any pain. You will probably be able to return to work after around a week.

THE RISKS

- **Bleeding/pain/swelling** These are easily treatable and usually temporary.
- **Necrosis** (See Glossary)
- **Scars** Some patients develop an unsightly scar that looks like an indentation around the wound site; surgeons call this a slot deformity.
- **Abnormal hair growth** Sometimes hair can grow in the wrong direction around the scar.
- **Numbness** It is possible that you will feel temporary or more persistent loss of sensation in the scalp.
- **Reaction to the anaesthetic** This complication is relevant to all surgery. Your pre-surgery consultation with your anaesthetist should lessen any likelihood of a reaction to the anaesthetic.

SCALP REDUCTION SURGERY

The scalp reduction operation involves removing strips of bald skin on the scalp of the patient, then stretching and stitching together adjacent hair-bearing sections. This operation is very limited in its scope if used alone, and so is usually used in combination with hair grafting, scalp extension or scalp expansion, which create more hair-bearing skin to cover what has been removed. It is only useful where the scalp skin is loose, since skin can be pulled a very small distance alone. Scalp reduction is usually reserved for patients who have very advanced hair loss, as part of a combination of procedures. You are a good candidate for this surgery is you have loose scalp skin, and good hair on the sides and back of your head.

THE OPERATION

After administering a local anaesthetic and probably a sedative to help you relax, the surgeon cuts the area of baldness on the head, pulls together the sections of hair-bearing skin left and stitches them together. This immediately covers more of the head with hair, so it has pretty dramatic results. The normal size of the section that can be removed at any one time is around 3–4cm (1¼–1½ inches) wide. This operation is normally performed with a local anaesthetic, so you should go home the same day.

THE RECOVERY PROCESS

When you wake up from the operation, you will have a bandage strapped to your head. For the next couple of days, you can expect some headache, bruising and swelling. Your head will probably also feel quite numb, but this should pass. There will be a scar in the middle of your head, which will take a week or two to heal.

THE RISKS

- **Bleeding, pain and swelling** These are easily treatable and usually temporary.
- **Scars** Scalp reductions leave large scars on the scalp. The scarring is the reason why this is a procedure not normally carried out on its own.
- **Scalp stretch** The scalp skin can stretch after the operation, eventually returning to its pre-operation position, which can create unsightly loose skin on the scalp. When this happens, some patients report that the bald spot looks larger than before.
- **Numbness** It is possible to feel temporary or more persistent loss of sensation in the scalp.
- **Reaction to the anaesthetic** This complication is relevant to all surgery. Your pre-surgery consultation with your anaesthetist should lessen any likelihood of a reaction to the anaesthetic.

SCALP EXPANSION

This is very similar to the above, but surgeons insert small inflatable balloons under the hair-bearing skin on the scalp and gently inflate them to create more hair-bearing skin, which can mean a rather unsightly profile for the patient for a time. Once the skin has stretched sufficiently over the balloons, they are removed and a scalp reduction procedure is performed utilizing the extra skin created.

SCALP EXTENSION

A scalp extension is a gruesome-sounding procedure whereby a device with rows of little hooks connected by elastic bands is placed under the skin during a scalp reduction procedure. Over four weeks, tension on the bands begins to stretch the scalp skin, which allows for a further scalp reduction utilizing the excess skin that has been created. A scalp extension is generally thought to be slightly less uncomfortable and certainly less unsightly than a scalp expansion. However, it doesn't create as much new hair-bearing skin as the expansion, so may take longer to see results.

THE ALTERNATIVES

This is one area where a fear of the scalpel will still leave you with plenty of options. Nowadays there are over-the-counter drug treatments for baldness and also prescription medicines, some of which have been extensively tested and have produced good results in some patients. In recent years, laser treatment for hair loss has advanced considerably, and even wigs and hairpieces are much improved today.

> **DID YOU KNOW?**
> The average human head has 120,000 hairs on it.

IN SHORT

Hair restoration surgery has come a long way from the first operations performed in the thirties. There are now a number of surgical options. Though scalp lifting is at present mainly only used for trauma victims, it nevertheless is an option to consider. Scalp reduction surgery, particularly when used in conjunction with scalp extension or scalp expansion, can provide a permanent and reliable hair covering. The most exciting developments in this field are undoubtedly the hair transplanting procedures that graft hair follicles from the hair-bearing skin to the bald parts of the scalp. Surgeons are becoming so skilled in this procedure that a natural look is now an achievable possibility.

The risks associated with this branch of surgery are minimal and discomfort levels are manageable, even if some of the skin-stretching systems can be rather unsightly while they work. Advances in technique ensure that now more than ever a bespoke solution can be created for every patient. As always, proceed with caution. Opt for surgery only when you have fully researched all of the suitable treatments, have been fully briefed and are completely happy to continue. In general, hair restoration surgery is a reliable solution for baldness and the results can dramatically and instantly improve self-esteem.

CONTOURING FACIAL FAT

As we age, the skin on our face becomes thinner and the underlying muscles weaker, which results in the familiar ageing process we all undergo. Sometimes a facelift is not the answer to the problem – it may be that all we need to restore a youthful look is a little nipping and plumping. But be warned: altering the contours of the face is a delicate business. More often than not it requires a combination of procedures to achieve the desired effect. If this is you, one subtle rejuvenating technique that you might consider effective is the fat transfer.

While liposuction (page 115) streamlines body shape through removing fat with a metal cannula (hollow tube), *microliposuction* (page 116) does the same for the face but in far smaller quantities. However, removing fat from the face is not always enough to create the desired effect. Sometimes surgeons will carry out a procedure that transfers fatty cells taken from elsewhere in the body into other areas of the face to redistribute fat and plump out those contours that feel the effects of time most acutely. This is called the *fat transfer*.

CONSIDERING SURGERY

Fat transfer is a surgical procedure that removes fat from a donor site in the body, most often the thighs, buttocks, abdomen or knees, and injects it into the face to add more volume. It is often combined with chin implants (page 76), cheek implants (page 83), ablative laser skin resurfacing (page 245) or chemical peels (page 231), which are all treatments to rejuvenate the face, plumping out wrinkles and crow's feet and smoothing the skin. Sometimes it is also used in other parts of the body to add volume to areas that lack fat, which can happen after excessive liposuction.

THE OPERATION

Your surgeon removes the fat from the donor area deep in the subcutaneous layer of skin via a small incision into which a small metal cannula is inserted. This fat is normally washed and then injected into the face using a series of tiny needles. If the fat is being injected elsewhere in the body, a larger needle may be used.

THE RECOVERY PROCESS

How long it takes you to get over the op largely depends on the extent of the procedure. You can expect that your face will become swollen. This should resolve over the course of a couple of weeks. Itching is not uncommon, and the area might feel tight as a result of the swelling for about a week. You'll look pretty bruised at first. This may take a couple of weeks to pass. The result of the fat transfer will only properly be seen after a couple of months. You can help yourself recover by resting for the first forty-eight hours after the procedure, preferably on propped-up pillows in bed. Try to use your facial muscles as little as possible during this time – no laughing and not too much talking. Recovery is a serious business! Don't get the wounds wet during the first week, and slowly increase your activity after the second week. Try not to touch the area where the fat has been injected, as it could leave permanent marks. Avoid strenuous exercise for about three weeks and try not to do anything that will increase the blood pressure in your head, such as bending or lifting, for a couple of weeks. If you experience pain, take painkillers as directed by your surgeon. If you notice any signs of infection, pain or discharge, contact your surgeon immediately.

THE RISKS

Fat transferring is not an exact science, and it relies heavily on the skill of the individual surgeon. Facial nerve injury is a potential complication, and you do run the risk of lumpiness and some discoloration if the procedure doesn't go smoothly. As with all surgical procedures, the operation site can become infected but this is rare. It is normally treated with antibiotics should it occur.

IN SHORT

A fat transfer is a procedure that surgeons use to alter the contours of the face. During the procedure, your surgeon will remove fat from a donor site on your body and inject small quantities into the face to soften wrinkles and plump out cheeks. The fat will not be rejected since it is your own. This procedure is often used in combination with other contouring procedures, such as chin or cheek implants or laser skin resurfacing, in order to build a dramatic overall result. Although generally very safe, it relies heavily on the skill of the surgeon. You'll feel bruised and swollen after the op, but you should be back on your feet pretty quickly. As always proceed with caution. Opt for the procedure only when you have fully researched all of the suitable treatments, have realistic expectations of what surgery can achieve, have been fully briefed and are completely happy to continue. In general, fat transfer is a simple solution to redefine the contours of the face and the results can be dramatic for what is essentially minimal discomfort.

FREQUENTLY ASKED QUESTIONS

Q Will I have to stay in hospital?

A This depends on the procedures you are having done at one time. Performed on its own, the fat transfer procedure is carried out under a light general anaesthetic and doesn't require you to stay overnight.

Q How long does it take?

A Since the operation is performed in two parts, a fat transfer procedure normally takes around two hours. However, it is most often performed in combination with other procedures, which would mean a much longer operation time.

Q How long will the results last?

A Approximately 30–40 per cent of fat cells transferred by this technique are expected to survive permanently. The remainder will die and be absorbed by the body. This process will take two to three months, so it is after this period that what you see is what you get. Different areas have a better fat cell survival than others – for example, cheeks are better than lips.

Q What can fat transfer do?

A Transferring fat from other parts of your body to your face can improve wrinkles, soften crow's feet and laughter lines and plump out sunken cheeks. It can also soften the appearance of some facial scars.

Q What can't a fat transfer do?

A This procedure does not resurface the skin, nor can it address jowls or a saggy neck. These conditions are better treated with a facelift.

Q What are the alternatives?

A Other procedures that can have a rejuvenating effect on the face include the thread lift (page 275), chemical peels (page 231), botulinum toxin injections (page 299), dermal fillers (page 281), autologous cell therapy (page 290), ablative laser skin resurfacing (page 245) and fractional laser skin resurfacing (page 263).

COSMETIC SURGERY:
THE BODY

Cosmetic surgery for the body is serious surgery which requires
a commitment to aftercare and a realistic attitude, but which
can provide you with a dramatic transformation. Whether you're
considering these procedures to reconstruct your body after multiple
pregnancies or massive weight loss, or are merely more interested
in the latest in buttock implants, this section will give you the
information you'll need to get prepared and recover as quickly and
successfully as possible. After a look at what liposuction can do for
stubborn fat, we move on to an in-depth chapter on probably the
most popular area for bodily surgical enhancement: the breasts.
We'll even discuss surgery for the penis, vagina and labia, so there's
literally no body part that will be left uncovered!

LIPOSUCTION

We've all got those extra lumps and bumps on our bodies where we store fat. For most women, it's around the hips and thighs, while for men it's around the middle. The good news is that cosmetic surgery has come up with a way of ironing out some of the more unsightly contours of your body. The bad news is that it's not a magic wand to make you thin, as many people still believe it is.

The only way permanently to maintain a healthy figure is to follow a balanced diet backed up by regular exercise. This hasn't changed and probably never will. What has changed is that medical science can now supplement your own hard work by literally sucking out the most stubborn fat that no amount of exercise or diet can shift, in order to streamline your silhouette a little further.

ABOUT LIPOSUCTION

Liposuction is a surgical procedure to remove fatty deposits that are resistant to diet and exercise. It can be performed in a variety of places on the body, but most often is used to treat the thighs, tummy, knees, arms, neck and back. Although it is a straightforward procedure that can have dramatic results, there are many limitations on how the treatment can be used. The more fat is removed, the greater the trauma to the body. Therefore, removing large amounts of fat from the body would simply be too risky. The body would be subject to shock, and a stay in intensive care and a blood transfusion might be necessary. That would be against one of the main principles of cosmetic surgery: do no harm.

Microliposuction is essentially the same procedure applied to the face, but the volume of fat removed is obviously much smaller than for the body, and much finer instruments are used. Microliposuction is sometimes combined with fat transfer (page 108), to redistribute the fat in the face along more aesthetic contours.

ABOUT FAT

Like it or loathe it, as humans we need some fat to help us store energy in our body. Fat plays a vital role in maintaining our hair and skin, protecting our internal organs and maintaining body temperature, and this fat distribution is genetically predetermined. When we take in more fat than we need, the body stores the extra fat in the fat cells, causing them to enlarge, just in case we need the fat in the future. Unfortunately, we do not always store the fat evenly and it is this that leads to the localized areas of flab that we find so unappealing. As we get older, we store more body fat because our metabolism slows down and we tend to be less active. The layer where this fat is stored is called the subcutaneous fatty tissue, and this, along with the deeper layers beneath it, is where liposuction is performed.

BEFORE LIPOSUCTION Your surgeon will advise you to stop taking aspirin or anti-inflammatory tablets and vitamin E. This is to reduce the likelihood of bleeding after the operation.

THE SURGERY

Though there are many variations on technique, the basic procedure for liposuction remains the same. The surgeon makes a number of small incisions in the skin near the area where the fat is to be removed. A relatively large volume of saline solution is infused into the area to make the tissues stiff and cause the small blood vessels to constrict. The surgeon then inserts a cannula (a sort of hollow metal tube) into the incision, burrowing into the fatty tissue. Once the surgeon has broken up the fat in the area, it will be drawn from the body using a large syringe or a suction machine connected to the cannula by a tube. The operation removes fat cells only; no blood vessels, nerves or other tissues are removed. Your surgeon will take care to leave just the right amount of fat to prevent hollowing out or dimpling, while removing as much fat as possible. The incision marks are then stitched up, and dressings placed over the wounds.

WHERE LIPOSUCTION CAN BE DONE ON THE BODY

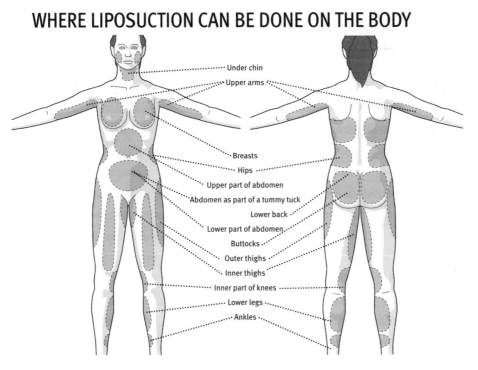

Under chin
Upper arms
Breasts
Hips
Upper part of abdomen
Abdomen as part of a tummy tuck
Lower back
Lower part of abdomen
Buttocks
Outer thighs
Inner thighs
Inner part of knees
Lower legs
Ankles

TYPES OF LIPOSUCTION

There are many ways in which the liposuction technique has been adapted in order to make it safer, less invasive and more straightforward. The main types of liposuction are shown in the following chart:

NAME	WHAT IT INVOLVES	ADVANTAGES/DISADVANTAGES	WHO IS MOST SUITABLE
Wet liposuction	The surgeon injects about the same amount of fluid as the amount of fat to be removed into the area to be treated, before suctioning the fat with a blunt metal cannula. This is done to reduce the likelihood of bleeding and to loosen the fat cells to be removed.	This is the technique most widely used by surgeons at the moment. It is the preferred method of liposuction if a large amount of fatty tissue is to be removed.	Anyone who is suitable for liposuction; depends on the surgeon's preference.
Tumescent liposuction	Essentially a wet liposuction, the surgeon injects a very large amount of tumescent solution of saline and adrenalin into the area to be treated. The amount injected is usually about two or three times as much as the amount to be removed.	The tumescent solution makes the fat easier to remove and reduces the likelihood of bleeding. This procedure is usually preferred if the procedure is carried out under local anaesthesia only.	Anyone who is suitable for liposuction; depends on the surgeon's preference.
Power-assisted liposuction	The surgeon uses a special cannula that is rotated by a small motor in the instrument handle.	Since the surgeon doesn't have to break up the fat through his own hand movements, this procedure is usually more comfortable for the surgeon. There is no advantage in terms of the result, and the procedure is more expensive because of the costly equipment.	Anyone who is suitable for liposuction; depends on the surgeon's preference and whether the surgeon has the equipment.

Ultrasound liposuction	As part of the preparation of the area, the surgeon uses ultrasound to break up the fat cells to be removed.	This can be a more effective technique and is usually reserved for difficult areas of the body to treat, such as the back, but you'll be in surgery for longer with this procedure. You'll also be at a greater risk of burning and fluid collecting under the skin.	Usually reserved for previous liposuction corrections or for patients with particularly dense fat tissue.
External ultrasound liposuction	Instead of using an internal ultrasound, the waves are transmitted into the body without making an incision. The fat is removed by a standard liposuction cannula.	Fairly new, this procedure has not been used a great deal yet, though it is believed to be less painful for the patient and it allows surgeons to treat large areas at a time. It is, however, more time-consuming, and the results are no better than standard liposuction.	Anyone who is suitable for liposuction; depends on the surgeon's preference.
External ultrasound liposuction	The cannula used is the size of a needle.	This technique is reserved for facial liposuction, where very small deposits of fat are removed to great effect.	Anyone who is suitable for facial liposuction.
Liposculpture	This technique uses a cannula attached to a large syringe, which produces the suction needed to remove fat.	The procedure is used mostly under local anaesthesia. The results are comparable with other techniques, but it is very time-consuming.	Anyone who wants liposuction under local anaesthesia.

STAYING IN HOSPITAL

The length of hospitalization depends on the type of liposuction you have and how much fat is taken. In general, the smaller the amount of fat reduced, the more likely you are to have the procedure as a day case. Most surgeons are happy to remove up to $3\frac{1}{2}$ litres (6 pints) of fat for a day case. For anything more, you'll be losing so much fluid that you will have to be monitored to see if you need a blood transfusion, which will mean an overnight stay. In my opinion, 4 litres (7 pints) in a session is a maximum – but at this amount, the chances of complications are increased. During the operation the surgeon will also measure the amount of fat that is removed from each area so that he is able to maintain symmetry around the body.

WHAT HAPPENS DURING RECOVERY?

You'll come round from the operation feeling sore and swollen, but you shouldn't be in too much pain. You'll be swaddled in a pressure garment over the wounds and you'll have to wear this for the next few weeks to prevent fluid from collecting around the treatment site. Before you go home, you'll be told how to wash and how to look after your wounds. If you have had a general anaesthetic, you'll need to have enlisted the support of someone sympathetic to help you while you get over the anaesthetic. They'll need to drive you home. You'll be on your feet again twenty-four to forty-eight hours after the procedure.

At home, you can help recovery by walking as much as possible to prevent any thrombosis (blood clot) in your legs. You can take painkillers, should you need to, as directed by your surgeon. Any stitches will be removed seven to ten days later. You'll probably be told that you can't do any strenuous exercise for around a month. When you are able to go back to work will depend on how much fat was taken away. At most, it'll be about ten days that you need to have off. Remember that swelling and bruising can take a number of weeks, even months, to settle, so you won't have an idea of your results for at least a couple of months after surgery.

THE RISKS

Liposuction is major surgery that should not be entered into lightly. Though considered safe, there are a number of possible complications:

- **Scars** Liposuction scars are very fine and short. They'll be easily noticeable at first, but they should fade with time. It is rare for them to become unsightly.
- **Infection** With liposuction, the infection rate is very small.
- **Haematoma/Seroma** (See Glossary)
- **Numbness/nerve damage** Some patients find that there is a loss of sensation around the treatment site. It is normal for this to persist for a few months after liposuction, but it can be permanent.
- **Unfavourable result** Liposuction is not an exact science. Your surgeon will try to remove as much fat as possible, as evenly as possible, but he will only remove an amount that is safe. It is important that you have realistic expectations of what surgery can achieve.
- **Skin changes** Skin can become lumpy or ripply after liposuction. It may also lose its natural colour and the pigment can change, too.
- **Blood clots** Problematic blood clotting is more likely if leg liposuction has been performed, though surgeons will generally put in place every precaution to prevent this from occurring.
- **Burns** There is a risk of burning from ultrasound-assisted liposuction, though this is rare.
- **Fat embolism syndrome** In the twenty-five or so years that liposuction has been in use, there have been a few cases where fat has entered the bloodstream after liposuction. If this happens,

it can prove fatal. Having said this, I have never seen it
during my experience, nor heard of it other than the occasional
reported case. With an experienced practitioner, it is very unlikely
indeed.

- **Reaction to the anaesthetic** This complication is relevant to
  all surgery. Your pre-surgery consultation with your
  anaesthetist should lessen any likelihood of a reaction to the
  anaesthetic.

IN SHORT

A number of types of liposuction can be employed to remove
stubborn fatty deposits from the body. Essentially a surgeon will
make several short incisions, insert a cannula and break up the fatty
tissue before removing it via suction. Surgeons are becoming more
and more skilled in this procedure, and, using microliposuction, it
is now possible to remove even tiny amounts of fat from the face to
provide a finer contour.

The risks associated with this procedure are very small, and
discomfort levels are certainly manageable. However, liposuction
is not a substitute for a healthy diet, since it can only remove fat
that is resistant to exercise. If you ask a surgeon for liposuction in
the belief that it will make you thin, you will almost certainly be
turned away. As always proceed with caution. Opt for surgery only
when you have fully researched all of the suitable treatments, have
been fully briefed and are completely happy to continue. In general,
liposuction is a reliable solution to treat stubborn flab, and the
results can dramatically and instantly improve a patient's self-
esteem.

FREQUENTLY ASKED QUESTIONS

Q How long has liposuction been around?

A The first surgeon to describe using a cannula, which is a long, thin, tubular instrument, to remove fat is believed to have been the Frenchman Charles Dujarrier, working in the twenties. Unfortunately, his primitive attempts at liposuction proved disastrous. For this reason, the technique was largely abandoned until the sixties. Once revived, liposuction was performed solely in Europe until the eighties, when American surgeons began to show an interest again. Since then, demand for the procedure has risen dramatically.

Q How long does it take?

A This largely depends on how much fat is being removed and how. Liposuction typically takes anywhere between one and three hours to complete. Ask your surgeon about your own case.

Q What can liposuction do?

A Liposuction can permanently rid you of the areas of your body where fat accumulates: say goodbye to huge saddlebags, fat knees and flabby arms.

Q What can't liposuction do?

A Liposuction will not make you thin. It cannot be used as a substitute for a healthy diet and plenty of exercise if you are overweight. Nor will it get rid of cellulite, stretch marks or excess skin. It's a specific treatment for a localized problem, not a shortcut to a size ten.

Q Is there anyone who is unsuitable for liposuction?

A If you are a fairly young and generally healthy person with localized fat deposits on your body, you are a good candidate for liposuction. If you are a bit older but reasonably close to a healthy weight, you may also be a suitable candidate. If you are in your teens, liposuction is not for you; your weight still hasn't really settled yet, and so liposuction would not achieve what you want. If you have a blood disorder that requires you to take anticoagulants, or you suffer from heart disease or diabetes, the risk of complications after surgery is probably too high to merit the procedure.

Ⓠ How common is the operation?

Ⓐ This is probably the most commonly performed cosmetic surgical procedure. In the United States in 2005, over 450,000 people had liposuction.

Ⓠ What are the alternatives?

Ⓐ Since liposuction is not a way of getting slimmer, a healthy diet and a good exercise routine to shift a few excess pounds could actually provide the change in body shape you are looking for. Your surgeon will probably want to know that you have at least tried to diet and exercise the stubborn fat away before he'll consider you for surgery anyway. For those whose problem is not so much localized fat, but more of a post-baby belly, then a tummy tuck (page 175) is probably worth looking into.

THE BREASTS

If you are female, your breasts are perhaps the most obvious sign of your sexuality. We all know that they come in all shapes and sizes, but few women are completely happy with their breasts, perceiving them as too small, too big, too droopy or maybe just a bit of a strange shape. Many women consider their breasts essential to their femininity, and so any perceived idiosyncrasy can be unwelcome. Breast surgery is one of the most popular cosmetic procedures available – certainly it is the body surgery that I perform most often – and, increasingly, this is becoming an operation many younger women seek.

ABOUT YOUR BREASTS

Your breasts are made of fibrous connective tissue, fat and milk-producing glands. The amount of each differs for every woman, which is why everyone's breasts are so different. The weight of your breasts is supported by a system of ligaments that connect the chest wall to the skin, while the fat in your breasts makes them stick out. The areola (the skin around the nipple) is dotted with small lumps, which are oil-producing glands that keep it moist. Inside the breast, resting alongside the fat and fibrous tissue, there are around fifteen to twenty-five glands called lobes. These contain alveoli, which produce the milk. The lobes are connected to the nipple via a system of ducts that converge and open at the nipple. It is this glandular part of the breast that responds to the hormonal cycle and causes the changes associated with menstruation and pregnancy.

WHY YOUR BREASTS SAG

There are a number of ways in which your breasts change throughout life, all of which eventually begin to take their toll on the ligaments that support your breasts.

- **Menstrual cycle** Each month your breasts go through their own cycle, which is directly related to menstruation. Once you ovulate, the blood supply to the breasts increases. They begin to retain this fluid and your chest begins to swell. Eventually, if the egg that has been released isn't fertilized, hormone levels fall and your breasts return to normal.

- **Pregnancy** If the egg is fertilized after ovulation, there is an increase in oestrogen in the body and the blood supply increases to the breast even further. By the time you have your baby, your breasts are around twice their normal size. Once breastfeeding has finished, your breasts will once again return to their original size. However, the ligaments that support your breasts have now been permanently stretched.

- **Hormone factors** The contraceptive pill, HRT and the menopause all affect your breasts, too, causing them to swell or shrink accordingly.

- **Weight gain and loss** The breasts can increase or reduce in size in line with your weight because so much of your breast is made up of fat.

- **Ageing** The ligaments that support the weight of your breasts naturally get weaker with age, reducing their ability to hold the breasts in their natural position relatively high on the chest wall.

Considering the changes your breasts have to put up with every month, every baby and every year, are you really surprised that they begin to look a little weary after your fortieth birthday?

CONSIDERING SURGERY

Because breasts are extremely varied, so are the operations and procedures involved in altering their shape. The general medical term for breast procedures is *mammaplasty*. The bad news is that virtually all mammaplasty procedures cause scarring that you'll be able to see on the breasts themselves. Unless you have implants inserted via your armpit, there will be scars under the crease of your breast, around the areola, and possibly running from the areola to the scar under the crease. Also, for many operations, your ability to breastfeed could be restricted. Consider all this carefully before you head into the operating theatre.

BREAST AUGMENTATION

Breast augmentation is one of the most popular cosmetic surgery procedures, and one that I perform between eighty to a hundred times a year. If you are unhappy with your breasts because you feel they're not big enough, or you are unhappy about their shape, you can take some comfort from the fact that you are certainly not alone.

Women who choose to have a breast augmentation may have considered surgery because they feel their breasts are too small or are noticeably different in size, or they may have shrunk after pregnancy or losing weight, or merely have dropped or shrivelled with age. Some augmentation operations are also carried out to correct developmental defects such as Poland's syndrome (where the breast and its underlying muscle fail to grow) or for reconstructive purposes, such as those following mastectomy.

WHAT ARE IMPLANTS MADE OF? Breast implants are made of a silicone outer layer, which can be either smooth or textured. The implant is filled with silicone gel or saline (salt water). A few years ago, alternative implants containing soya bean oil or hydrogel were promoted, but their use in the UK has now been discontinued because of fears over safety.

THE OPERATION

Breast augmentation involves placing an implant either under your breast tissue, or under your breast tissue and muscle, in order to increase the size of your breasts. The operation varies considerably but, essentially, cuts will be made around the breast to allow access underneath. From here, the surgeon creates a pocket for the implant and places it in that pocket. The incision is then closed with stitches. There are a number of options to consider when you and your surgeon plan your breast augmentation operation, so make sure you discuss everything thoroughly before your proceed. Nowadays there are so many variables that surgeons are in a position to create a bespoke operation for each patient. In a nutshell, your choices fall into three categories: type of implant, site of incision and placement of the implant pocket.

CHOOSING THE RIGHT IMPLANT

Your first choice is about the type of implant you are opting for:

The right size To help you decide what size you want to be, buy a bra you would like to fill and fill it with tissues or socks. You can then see how it is going to look in proportion to the rest of your chest and body. You might find that taking this bra to your consultation helps, as most patients have an idea of how large they would like to be by this stage. However, there are limitations to the size, and if you go to a consultation with an unreasonable request many surgeons will choose not to operate. Very large implants, and the operation to insert them, have their problems. The operation is not about stuffing any size of implants into a pocket – there are practical long-term considerations, as well as aesthetic ones. For surgeons, the most accurate way to measure the volume necessary to produce the desired change in cup size is by using an inflatable implant and measuring its volume, before choosing the right size of implant.

The right shape It is possible to choose between teardrop-shaped and round implants. Though each surgeon has their own preferences, in my practice I do not use teardrop implants because they can only be inserted through a very large incision in the breast fold, owing to the fact that these implants are very stiff and will not pass through a normal-sized incision. Therefore, my own preference is to use round implants.

About silicone Modern silicone implants have a thick and sturdy outer shell of several layers of silicone rubber that encases a semi-solid silicone gel. Years ago, this outer layer wasn't very thick and was prone to rupture, but modern implants are much thicker and therefore less likely to split. If the implant does rupture, the scar tissue that your body will have built up around the implant generally holds the silicone gel in place anyway. Silicone gel has a similar feel to body fat. This makes the implant look and feel more natural as it is soft and malleable.

IS SILICONE SAFE? Silicone implants were the implant of choice from their introduction in the sixties until the early nineties, when their safety was called into question by a group of American lawyers. They claimed that there was a link between implants and breast cancer, and between implants and birth defects in children born to mothers with implants. This was followed by another claim that there was also a link between silicone breast implants and connective tissue disorders such as rheumatoid arthritis, systemic lupus erythematosus and myalgic encephalitis (ME). The claims described a frightening complication in women whose implants had ruptured, leading to migration of the silicone to other parts of the body. As a result, silicone implants were banned for use in cosmetic enhancements in the United States from 1992 until 2006.

However, on the basis of large trials in the United States, it has since been agreed that silicone implants have nothing to do with breast cancer or developmental birth defects, and, in fact, the evidence currently available suggests that women with implants actually have a lower rate of breast cancer. In 1999, scientists from the Institute of Medicine in the United States published a detailed report on breast implants. Their research concluded that there is no scientific evidence of a connection between breast implants and any autoimmune disease. Research continues, but the Department of Health in the UK has never seen fit to ban silicone implants. Many UK doctors believe that silicone remains the best choice for implants today.

About saline Saline implants are made of a thick and sturdy silicone outer shell, but the filler content of the implant is a salt and water mixture. These implants are normally filled with the saline solution only after the implant itself has been inserted into the body. When the filling tube is withdrawn, the valve in the outer shell closes. Since the saline implant is small when inserted, the incision needed is smaller than for a silicone implant.

The implants come in different sizes ranging from around 150 cubic cm (9 cubic inches) to over 600 cubic cm (36 cubic inches), thus allowing the surgeon to adjust the volume in each implant. This means that the surgeon can easily balance a discrepancy in size between the breasts.

However, saline implants are generally considered to feel less natural than silicone gel implants. They also have a greater tendency to wrinkle, which can sometimes be seen, particularly in very thin women. The implant itself is more likely to leak and deflate than silicone. Around 10 per cent of saline implants deflate. When this happens the breast deflates quickly and the implant will need to be replaced, although the saline filling is not harmful to the body and so will quickly and easily be absorbed. Very few implant patients, knowing the facts of saline vs. silicone, insist on saline implants, but the decision should be nevertheless carefully considered before you continue.

INCISION LOCATION OPTIONS

No matter where you choose to have the incisions for the implants, you will have scars, but they should fade over time. These are the options:

Transaxilliary The surgeon will insert the implant via an incision in your armpit. This approach produces the most natural result, though it is technically very demanding. When the scar has faded it is virtually imperceptible. This is my own preferred method.

Periareolar The incision is made around the lower half of the dark circle of your nipple (the areola). The surgeon cuts through the breast tissue, and then creates the pocket. The scars are usually thin, as the skin around your nipple heals very well.

Inframammary This is the approach favoured by most surgeons because of its ease. It involves making an incision in the crease underneath the breast. Access is easy but the scars are longer.

Transumbilical The surgeon makes an incision in your belly button, before burrowing under the skin up to the breasts. This is a complicated procedure that can only be used for saline implants, but it can provide good results in the right patient and with an experienced surgeon.

POCKET PLACEMENT OPTIONS

Once you have decided which implant and where the scar will be, you and your surgeon have one more decision to make. There are two options as to where the implant can rest in the body:

Submuscular augmentation Here, the implants rest behind both the breast tissue and the pectoralis muscle in the chest. This is the preferred location in around 80 per cent of patients who undergo breast augmentation, mainly because it allows for an extra layer of protection for the implant and is thought also to reduce the likelihood of hard scar tissue forming. I recommend this approach because it produces a much more natural result.

Subglandular augmentation The implants are inserted above the chest muscle, but underneath the breast tissue. This method may benefit you if you are concerned about saggy breasts, as the implants can be placed a little lower, creating a slightly more natural shape. This procedure is also less painful than the under-muscle alternative. However, placing the implant above the muscle makes it more likely that you will be able to feel the implant, and any wrinkling can be more obvious.

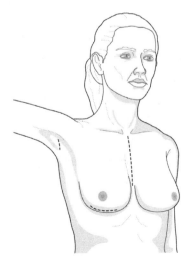

Incision location options for breast augmentation

THE RECOVERY PROCESS

When you wake up from the operation you may have pain and your chest will be strapped. There will be drains close to the wound site to relieve any fluid that collects in the breast pocket; these drains will be removed before you leave hospital. A nurse will give you instructions about how to care for your breasts in the short and long term, which may or may not include instructions on massaging your breasts. You will leave the hospital wearing a soft sports bra.

When you get home from hospital, rest with your feet up for at least two days. Most patients find that they can go back to work after around two weeks. You may take recommended painkillers for any pain, as advised by your surgeon. Take extra care until your stitches are removed around a week after the operation.

Avoid wearing a wired bra for at least three weeks – continue to wear a soft bra for the first few weeks, as directed by your surgeon, to provide the breast with generous support. Do not use deodorant, and stick to unperfumed or uncoloured soap for the first few weeks. Move your arms with care, but keep your shoulder joints mobile. Do not do any heavy lifting for four weeks after surgery. Gradually increase your arm activity. It will be around six weeks before you can exercise again. Stick to sunscreen factor 25 in the future.

Contact the surgery if you experience severe pain, bruising, discharge from the wound or fever. You can expect the pain, swelling, tenderness and bruising to remain for the first few days, and there is the possibility of a burning sensation in the nipples for a few weeks, but this should disappear. Residual swelling should ease after four or five weeks.

THE RISKS

- **Capsule formation** Although breast implants are inserted via a small incision in the skin, they necessitate a larger cut inside the breast. The body responds to this cut and the presence of the implant by forming scar tissue around the pocket site. This scar tissue forms differently in every person. Very thick and hard scarring can lead to a shell forming around the implant, squeezing it into a hard ball, which can be painful and unsightly. This 'capsule' is thought to occur in as many as one in ten implant operations. In an attempt to combat it, many modern implants now have a rough outer texture which, it is claimed, can restrict the growth of scar tissue. If the capsule is significant it may require further surgery to enlarge the pocket and relieve pressure on the implant.
- **Leaking** Modern implants are more resistant than ever to rupturing. However, around 10 per cent of women still experience leaking from their implants, some time after surgery. In saline implants, this can lead to the breast deflating quickly, but with silicone the process is much slower. If a split occurs with a silicone implant, the silicone will generally not leak outside the scar tissue that encapsulates it. If your implant does leak, you can expect the breast to become softer or unnaturally hard, and the implant will have to be removed and replaced with a new one.
- **Scars** The scars from breast augmentation are hidden in your armpit, around the base of the nipple or under the natural crease of the breast. External scars can become red and raised, but this is uncommon. Talk to your surgeon if you are prone to problem scarring.
- **Asymmetry** All women have naturally asymmetrical breasts, but it is possible that implants could exaggerate this difference.
- **Infection** This is rare, but if it occurs it has to be treated with antibiotics. If the infection does not respond to antibiotics, removal of the implant may be necessary.

- **Loss of sensation** There is usually a temporary difference in skin and nipple sensation following breast augmentation but it can be permanent. All types of approach are subject to this complication.
- **Seroma** Occasionally fluid can build up around the operation site. This may have to be drained but it usually settles without further intervention.
- **Bleeding** This can occur after any operation but is not very common. The presence of clotted blood inside the breast pocket is undesirable and has to be dealt with by removing the clot and stopping the bleeding.
- **Reaction to the anaesthetic** This complication is relevant to all surgery. Your pre-surgery consultation with your anaesthetist should lessen any likelihood of a reaction to the anaesthetic.

IN SHORT

Breast augmentation is probably one of the most common types of cosmetic surgery carried out today. It is an effective and highly refined procedure that can dramatically improve your appearance. Silicone gel implants are widely used as a natural-feeling alternative to saline implants. The type of implant, incision location and position of the pocket are decisions that you must carefully consider in consultation with your surgeon. Before proceeding, your surgeon will also want to be clear about your motivations and expectations.

The operation is carried out under general anaesthetic, but you can expect to feel sore and to be in some pain when you wake up, particularly if you opt to have the implant placed underneath the muscles of your chest. Sensible aftercare is required to achieve optimal results with this operation. There are few contraindications to having a breast augmentation, though smokers are at a greater risk of complications and recovery will take longer.

Among the risks associated with the surgery are hardening of the breast, leakage and loss of sensation. So, as always, proceed with caution. Opt for surgery only when you have fully researched all of the suitable treatments, have been fully briefed and are completely happy to continue. In general, breast augmentation is a popular solution for people who are unhappy with the appearance of their breasts, and the results can dramatically change your look.

FREQUENTLY ASKED QUESTIONS

Q What can breast augmentation do?

A Breast augmentation can increase the size of your breasts within reason and improve shape, sometimes giving a lifting effect.

Q What can't breast augmentation do?

A It cannot lift already heavily sagging breasts. It would have to be combined with an uplift operation (page 139) to achieve the desired effect.

Q How long does the operation take?

A Breast augmentation takes between one and two hours.

Q Will I have to stay in hospital?

A Breast augmentation is normally carried out under a general anaesthetic, which means that you will normally stay in hospital overnight.

Q How long will the implants last?

A At the moment breast implants last for around ten years, although this varies with each individual. Some patients have found that their implants have lasted closer to twenty years. Be aware, however, that your breasts will continue to age in the normal way, and so unfortunately you'll still be susceptible to the sagging that comes with age.

Q Will the implant affect mammography?

A Yes, breast implants do interfere with the results obtained by a mammogram. Be sure to tell the nurse or radiographer that you have implants before an X-ray so that they can adjust the technique to allow the mammogram still to be taken.

Q How long has the operation been around?

A The history of breast implants is relatively short. The first implant operations were conducted in 1962, using silicone.

Q Can I breastfeed with implants?

A It is possible to have an augmentation and still be able to breastfeed after surgery.

Q What are the alternatives?

A For women whose goal is enlargement, there is a non-surgical option, in which a device is placed over the breast and then slight suction applied from within. This, in some patients, appears to increase the breast volume by up to one cup size. It must be worn for eleven hours a day for an extended period of time. Failing that, it's back to external pads and push-up bras if you want a more voluptuous look.

BREAST LIFT

If you are a woman who has had children, chances are you're familiar with the deflating feeling that occurs after breastfeeding. You'll probably also have noticed that as you get older, your breasts seem to be heading on a downward trajectory that cannot be halted by any number of press-ups or push-up bras. Perhaps one of your breasts is considerably larger than the other. The operation that surgeons perform to readdress this sagging or asymmetry of the breast is called *mastopexy*. In this procedure, which I perform around twenty times a year, breasts are lifted, nipples hoisted and skin tightened to produce more youthful-looking, altogether perkier breasts. It is often carried out in combination with either augmentation (page 128) or reduction (page 150).

WHY BREASTS SAG Over time, the tissue in your breast gets tired of the constant swelling and shrinking caused by menstruation, pregnancy and weight loss and gain. The fibres in the breast can no longer stretch and spring back as they did in your youth, and before long you'll find that your breasts, which used to keep your armpits company, now are best friends with your belly button.

CONSIDERING SURGERY

If you want your breasts uplifted, you're going to have scars on them. Many women, however, are willing to accept scars in exchange for being able to wear fashionable clothes and bikinis with pride. Nevertheless, it is important to be realistic in your expectations. The breasts you had in your twenties will never return, but what a breast lift can offer is a close comparison. The surgeon will remodel your breast via a number of incisions. He will remove excess skin, reposition the nipple higher and tighten the skin underneath the nipple. Depending on the degree of sagging and the amount of scarring you can accept, there are a number of options to choose from when considering which breast lift to have.

You might be considering a breast lift when actually the operation that will make your breasts look more normal is a combination of uplifting and either augmentation or reduction. For example, if your nipple is above the crease of your breast, there is little a lift procedure will do; instead, consider an augmentation to put volume back into the breast and restore a youthful shape. On the other hand, if your breasts are droopy because they are very bulky, then a reduction operation is the best choice.

TYPES OF MASTOPEXY

Inverted T-scar mastopexy This is the standard operation to lift the breast, used for very large breasts and extensive sagging. The surgeon makes three incisions: one around the areola (skin around the nipple), one under the crease of the breast and another in a vertical line from the areola to the crease incision. The surgeon removes the excess skin and tissue and repositions the nipple higher. The three scars are stitched together to form an anchor shape.

Crescent mastopexy This is an operation suitable for women who have subtle sagging and want their problem solved with minimal scarring. The surgeon removes the skin from an incision that runs about halfway around the areola. Sometimes breast implants are also inserted through these incisions if required. The procedure can raise the nipple very slightly or alter the direction in which the nipple points.

Doughnut mastopexy This is usually done for women with slightly more saggy breasts who want a lift and a breast enlargement at the same time. The surgeon cuts the skin and removes the tissue in order to tighten the skin and lift the nipple. With this procedure the scar runs completely around the areola. The nipple itself can be moved upwards by 2–4cm ($^3/_4$–1$^1/_2$ inches).

Vertical scar mastopexy ('lollipop' technique) Instead of making an incision under the crease of the breast, the surgeon removes the tissue and skin via the areola and vertical incision only. The technique tends to work better where there is a reasonably small amount of tissue to be removed, i.e. the breast is not very large, and the nipple does not have to be moved far.

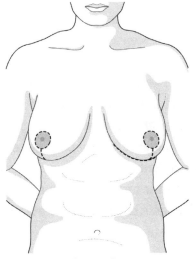

Location of scars for mastopexy

THE RECOVERY PROCESS

You will wake up from the operation feeling very swollen and sore, and you can expect this discomfort to last for the first few days after surgery. You are likely to have drainage tubes coming out from the skin to remove any excess fluid that may gather. You'll be given painkillers as required, which may or may not make you feel sick. You'll need to be able to rest at home for the first couple of days after surgery, and your surgeon will probably advise that you arrange for someone to be with you at all times for the first few days. You'll be instructed to wear a good-fitting soft bra for a number of weeks after surgery, to support your breasts while they settle. Try to avoid the temptation to disturb your dressing unless advised by your nurse. Also, avoid getting the scars wet, as that would increase your chance of infection. Your stitches will be removed one week after the procedure.

Most people find that they can go back to work after a week or so, though your surgeon will advise what is best for you: it may be substantially longer. You won't be allowed to drive for at least a week or lift heavy objects or do any exercise for around a month. Your breasts may feel tender for weeks or even months after the procedure. You could find that you have lost some sensation in your nipple or part of your breast for a while, but this should pass eventually.

Don't be surprised if initially the breasts look a strange shape and the nipples are puckered; this normally settles in a few months. Avoid sun exposure for at least three months – you'll be advised to use factor 25 sunscreen in the future. Scars don't completely settle until around a year after the operation. If you notice any signs of infection – e.g. your breasts become very warm to touch or you have a pus-like discharge, swelling, pain or fever – contact your surgeon immediately.

THE RISKS

There are a number of risks associated with a breast lift that are the same as for breast reduction. However, the risks are reduced with this procedure since it is less invasive. If you combine the lift with an augmentation, then, in addition to the above, remind yourself of the risks associated with implants. Before opting to have this procedure, be aware of the following:

- **Scars** The scars are designed to be undetectable while wearing a bikini top, though there is always scarring on the breasts themselves. Depending on the incisions, you may be left with a small scar around the nipple or a large anchor-type scar under the breast. At first, the scars will be red and lumpy, but they should fade to thin white lines with time. However, everyone heals differently and so the scars you get will depend on your general health and ability to heal.
- **Loss of sensitivity** Your nipple will probably lose some sensation after surgery. It is usually temporary, but sometimes it can be permanent.
- **Loss of the nipple** There is also a very small chance that you could lose your nipple altogether if the blood supply to the nipple is restricted during recovery. Talk to your surgeon about this – a new nipple can normally be created should this occur.
- **Asymmetry** It is possible that any difference in the size of your breasts might become more pronounced after surgery. If you feel that the difference is particularly bad, go back to your surgeon to discuss this.
- **Bleeding** It is unusual for bleeding to continue after surgery. Should this happen, however, you may have to be taken back to the operating theatre to stop the bleeding.
- **Infection** You may possibly get an infection after surgery. This is usually treated with antibiotics, which can delay the healing process.

- **Reaction to the anaesthetic** This complication is relevant to all surgery. Your pre-surgery consultation with your anaesthetist should lessen any likelihood of a reaction to the anaesthetic.

IN SHORT

The breast lift is an effective and highly refined procedure that can improve the appearance of your breasts through lifting the nipples and altering the position of the tissue around the nipples. Your surgeon will want to be clear about your motivations and expectations before proceeding. The operation itself is carried out under general anaesthetic, and you can expect to feel sore and to be in some pain when you wake up. Sensible aftercare is required to achieve optimal results with this operation. There are few reasons why you shouldn't have a breast reduction if you are fit and healthy. However, you might want to consider waiting until you have had a family, as there is no guarantee that you will be able to breastfeed following this operation. Among the risks associated with the surgery are scarring and loss of sensation. So, as always, proceed with caution. Opt for surgery only when you have fully researched all of the suitable treatments, have been fully briefed and are completely happy to continue. In general, a breast lift can be a solution for women who are unhappy with the appearance of their sagging breasts, and the results can leave you feeling a lot perkier!

FREQUENTLY ASKED QUESTIONS

Q Is there anyone who is unsuitable for a breast uplift?

A If your breast sag is a major concern to you, you have had your children and you are prepared for the scarring and recovery, you are probably a good candidate for the procedure. If you are yet to have children, consider postponing the operation as it may well affect your ability to breastfeed. If you are considering the operation because someone else has suggested it, then don't. This operation is a serious and irreversible procedure and it should be your decision alone to proceed.

Q How long does it take?

A Mastopexy takes around one to three hours.

Q Will I have to stay in hospital?

A The operation is carried out using a general anaesthetic, but you will probably be able to leave the hospital the same day or stay for just one night. Your surgeon will advise.

Q What can a breast lift do?

A A breast lift can reposition your breasts along a more youthful contour, often moving the nipple and reducing excess tissue at the same time.

Q What can't a breast lift do?

A A breast lift cannot raise the position of your breast on your chest wall. If the fold under your breast has also slipped downwards as a result of years of drooping, the lift you are left with may not be as high as you had hoped. A breast lift cannot give you back the firm tissue you had in your youth – it can only redress the existing tissue along a more youthful contour.

Q Can I breastfeed after lifting?

A Although never guaranteed, the mastopexy operation does not usually interfere with breastfeeding unless there has been a drastic alteration in sagging. However, further pregnancies will cause your breasts to swell again, which will make them sag again once you have finished breastfeeding.

Q How long will it last?

A Sadly, a breast lift is not permanent, since gravity will once again begin to affect the breast tissue that remains, the fibres will stretch and the breast will droop. However, the degree of sagging should be less. If you combine your breast lift with an augmentation, the weight of the implants may mean that you notice drooping again sooner than you had imagined you might. Weight gain, pregnancy and ageing will continue to affect your breasts in the normal way.

Q What are the alternatives?

A Once a breast has drooped and the skin and tissue have stretched, there is currently nothing else that can be done to restore a youthful contour other than surgery. A good supporting bra is the only prevention you can take against drooping.

NIPPLE RESHAPING

There are a minority of women whose nipples don't naturally protrude. The condition usually occurs in puberty but can occur at any time. These inverted nipples are generally caused by shortened milk ducts that pull the nipple back into the breast, and the condition is usually harmless.

If, however, your nipple suddenly becomes inverted, the first thing you should do is book an appointment with your GP. The sudden appearance of an inverted nipple could signify a number of other underlying conditions, and these need to be investigated further before surgery is considered. Should your doctor confirm that your problem is a harmless inversion, there is a short and simple surgical procedure that can correct the condition.

THE OPERATION

There are a variety of techniques that your surgeon might choose from. In the first, the surgeon will cut behind the nipple and free the nipple from the milk ducts that are pulling the nipple in. They will also place a stitch behind the nipple to try to prevent the nipple from dropping in again. This is the simplest way to make the nipple protrude. However, following this procedure, a very high proportion do drop back again. Another technique, which prevents recurrence of the nipple dropping back in, involves pulling a small island of nipple skin under the nipple to prevent it from slipping back. It is also possible for the surgeon to use a pin or a stud placed through the nipple during the healing phase until scar tissue is formed.

OTHER NIPPLE PROCEDURES

There are a few other procedures that surgeons use to reshape the nipple.

- To change the size or shape of the areola (the skin surrounding the nipple), particularly to reduce very large nipples, the surgeon will cut two circles on your breast: one around the circumference of the areola and one where the outer edge will be after surgery. The surgeon then removes the skin between the two lines and pulls the remaining skin and nipple together before stitching closed.

- A surgeon can make the nipple bigger by stretching the areola, though this is rarely done. Your surgeon can also transfer fat into the nipple to make it protrude further if desired.

- Some women's nipples can protrude excessively. If you feel that yours are too long and protrude too much, they can be made shorter by removing a segment from each nipple and reattaching it.

THE RISKS

The operation for inverted nipples is a minor procedure, but there is always a risk of complications. Aside from the general risks of surgery, such as infection, bleeding or a reaction to the anaesthetic, a specific risk is the possibility that you will lose some sensation in the nipple. Scarring is usually minimal, although in some individuals it may be a problem.

FREQUENTLY ASKED QUESTIONS

Q How long does it take?

A This procedure takes an hour.

Q Will I have to stay in hospital?

A You'll only need to have a local anaesthetic for this procedure and so be able to return home the same day.

Q What is recovery like?

A Other than having sore nipples, which may last for a couple of days, you'll be able to resume your normal activities almost straight away. There is virtually no scarring to contend with.

Q How long will the results of this operation last?

A The ducts will have been permanently severed, so the operation is generally permanent, although very rarely the condition can return.

Q Is there anyone who is unsuitable for these procedures?

A If you have inverted nipples and do not plan to breastfeed in the future, are generally in good health and are aware of the potential risks, you are a good candidate for this surgery. If you are yet to have children, you should probably leave this operation until you have had your family, as this surgery can prevent you from breastfeeding.

Q What are the alternatives?

A There is an alternative treatment to surgery, available on the high street, that uses a suction technique to pull the nipple out from the breast; however, the results are not always permanent. Surgery is the only permanent solution to the condition.

BREAST REDUCTION

If your breasts are significantly larger than the average, finding a bra to fit is probably the least of your worries. Breasts that are out of proportion with the rest of your body can be cumbersome, droopy and very uncomfortable. They can lead to backache, sore shoulders and even some skin conditions. And if you feel like your breasts have an impact on your psychological well-being, chances are you'll already have considered whether surgery can provide a solution.

Be warned, however: breast reduction surgery (also called *reduction mammaplasty*) is a major operation that should not be entered into lightly. That said, if you do suffer from the above problems, are unable to take part in sport and find it difficult to buy clothes that fit, you may wish to investigate a reduction mammoplasty via an initial consultation with your GP or a cosmetic or plastic surgeon.

DID YOU KNOW?
Surgeons have been refining breast reduction techniques for over a hundred years.

THE OPERATION

Breast reduction reduces the breast volume by removing breast tissue, fat and skin. The breasts are essentially cut to size, before being reshaped to form a new, smaller shape. Usually the nipple is repositioned and reduced. There are many ways in which your surgeon can operate, but all of the incisions available will form scars around the areola (dark skin around your nipple). The breast reduction may also be used to balance the size of your breasts with each other.

THE FIRST STEP: CONTACT YOUR GP Your GP will be able to advise you about your suitability for breast reduction surgery, since they know your medical history and, in particular, they know of any past operations or conditions that might affect how you recover. They will also be able to find out about whether you'd qualify for having this operation through the National Health Service. It is likely that as part of the qualification procedure you will be referred to both a surgeon and a psychologist or psychiatrist, who will assess your suitability further.

TYPES OF BREAST REDUCTION OPERATION

Standard breast reduction The surgeon will make three incisions: one around your areola, one under the crease of the breast and another in a vertical line from the areola to the breast crease. The surgeon will remove the excess skin and tissue and then reposition the nipple higher. The skin under the nipple is then stitched together to form an anchor shape.

Vertical scar breast reduction Instead of making an incision under the crease of the breast, the surgeon removes the tissue and skin via the areola and vertical incision only. The technique tends to work better on smaller breasts.

Breast reduction with nipple transfer Usually reserved for very large breasts, this operation involves the complete removal of the nipple before it is grafted back on to the breast. This may or may not take, and almost certainly all sensation will be lost.

Breast reduction with liposuction Because so much of the breast tissue is fat, the breasts can be reduced with liposuction only, but this is usually only possible when they are not saggy. (If you already have saggy breasts, then liposuction will probably make this more pronounced.) Liposuction can also be useful if treating very asymmetrical breasts.

WHAT ABOUT MAMMOGRAMS? Having this surgery does not interfere with the mammogram machine, so should you need to, you will be able to be screened for breast cancer in the normal way.

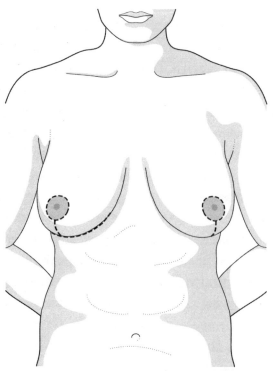

Locations of incisions for breast reduction

THE RECOVERY PROCESS

You will wake up from the operation feeling very swollen and sore, and you can expect this discomfort to last for the first few days after surgery. You are likely to have drainage tubes attached to the operation site, to remove any excess fluid that may gather. You'll be given painkillers as required, which may or may not make you feel sick. You'll need to be able to rest at home for the first couple of days after surgery, and your surgeon will probably suggest you arrange for someone to be with you at all times for the first few days. You'll be instructed to wear a good-fitting soft bra for a number of weeks after surgery, to support your breasts while they settle. Try to avoid the temptation to disturb your dressing unless advised by your nurse. Also, avoid getting the scars wet, as this would increase your chance of infection. Your stitches will be removed ten to fourteen days after the procedure.

Most people find that they can go back to work after a couple of weeks, though your surgeon will advise what is best for you: it may be longer. You won't be allowed to drive for at least a week, or to lift any heavy objects or do any exercise for around a month. Your breasts may feel tender and lumpy for weeks or even months after the procedure. You'll find that you can't really feel your nipple or part of your breast for a while, but this should pass eventually.

Don't be surprised if initially the breasts look a strange shape and the nipples are puckered; this normally settles in a few weeks. Avoid sun exposure for at least three months – you'll be advised to use factor 25 sunscreen in the future. The scars won't completely settle until around a year after the operation. If you notice any signs of infection – e.g. hot breasts, pus-like discharge, swelling, pain or fever – contact your surgeon immediately.

THE RISKS

There are a number of risks of surgery and consequences of the breast reduction operation that you should be aware of before opting to have this procedure:

- **Scars** The scars are designed to be undetectable while wearing a bikini top, though there is always scarring on the breasts themselves. Depending on the incisions, you may be left with a small scar around the nipple or a large anchor-type scar over the breast. At first, the scars will be red and lumpy, but they should fade to thin white lines with time. However, everyone heals differently and so the scars you get will depend on your general health and ability to heal. For the majority of women, the scars are an acceptable consequence of surgery to relieve their symptoms.

- **Inability to breastfeed** It is very rare for any woman to be able to breastfeed following breast reduction surgery, because during the operation the nipple is separated from the breast milk ducts. Young women should carefully consider this consequence before deciding to go ahead.

- **Loss of the nipple** Because the nipple is separated from some of the skin and tissue during the operation, there is a very small chance that you could lose your nipple altogether. Surgeons can normally create a new nipple should this occur.

- **Loss of sensitivity** Your nipple will probably lose some sensation after surgery. It is usually temporary, but sometimes it can be permanent.

- **Unfavourable result** It is very important that you discuss thoroughly with your surgeon beforehand the size of breasts you wish to achieve. There is no guarantee that you will end up with exactly the shape and size you want.

- **Asymmetry** It is possible that any difference in the size of your breasts might become more pronounced after surgery. If you feel that the difference is particularly bad, go back to your surgeon to discuss this.

- **Bleeding** Bleeding is controlled during surgery but some bleeding may continue after the operation, with blood collecting in the breast pocket. The bleeding may have to be stopped and the collected blood removed.
- **Infection** You may possibly get an infection after surgery. This is usually treated with antibiotics, which can delay the healing process.
- **Reaction to the anaesthetic** This complication is relevant to all surgery. Your pre-surgery consultation with your anaesthetist should lessen any likelihood of a reaction to the anaesthetic.

IN SHORT

Breast reduction is one of the few operations that may be available on the NHS. It is an effective and highly refined procedure that can reduce the weight, volume and shape of your breasts, but your surgeon will want to be clear about your motivations and expectations before proceeding. The operation itself is carried out under general anaesthetic, and you can expect to feel sore and to be in some pain when you wake up. Sensible aftercare is required to achieve optimal results.

There are few contraindications to having a breast reduction, but you might want to consider trying a diet to lose some body fat if you are overweight before you consider this procedure. Similarly, if you are young, have not yet had children and would like to breastfeed in the future, it could be advisable to wait for a few years as it is highly unlikely that you would be able to breastfeed after this operation. Among the risks associated with the surgery are scarring and loss of sensation. So, as always, proceed with caution. Opt for surgery only when you have fully researched all of the suitable treatments, have been fully briefed and are completely happy to continue. In general, breast reduction is a very reliable solution for people who are unhappy with the appearance of their large breasts, and the results can dramatically change your outlook.

FREQUENTLY ASKED QUESTIONS

Q Is there anyone who is unsuitable for breast reduction?

A Breast size changes with body weight, and so if your weight fluctuates, so will the size of your breasts. If your weight isn't stable, then it is unlikely that your GP or surgeon will recommend this procedure. Similarly, if you are particularly young, your surgeon and GP will probably advise you to wait until your breasts have stopped growing and you've had your family before having this surgery.

Q How common is the operation?

A More than 150,000 women in the United States had breast reductions in 2005. I perform this operation around twenty to forty times a year.

Q How long does it take?

A You'll be on the operating table for between two and four hours.

Q What can breast reduction do?

A Breast reduction can reduce the size and volume of your breasts, move your nipple or increase the symmetry of your breasts, thus reducing some of the uncomfortable symptoms associated with large breasts.

Q What can't the operation do?

A A breast reduction cannot guarantee that your breasts will be entirely symmetrical.

Q How long will the results of the operation last?

A Unless the operation is done when you are young and your breasts are still growing, there should never be any major increase in size after the operation. The two caveats to these are pregnancy, which causes the breasts to swell temporarily, and natural weight gain. If you put on a few stone, your breasts will get bigger as a result. Also, because all breasts droop with age, the fact that you have had your breasts reduced will not stop this.

Q What are the alternatives?

A If your large breasts are caused in part by the fact that you are also overweight, you may well find that if you dieted to a healthy weight, your breasts would also reduce in size. If you are not overweight, then other than learning to love your breasts or wearing a very good minimizer bra, there is little else that can be done.

MALE BREAST REDUCTION

If you're a man who has enlarged breast tissue, known in medical terms as gynaecomastia, there could be a number of reasons for its presence. In many, the existence of breast tissue is simply down to a weight problem, while in others it could point to an underlying genetic condition or hormone disorder. In all cases, it is likely to be embarrassing for the bearer, and the cause of some distress. Luckily, there are surgical procedures that can be employed to reduce male breast tissue. However, it should be considered only when your GP and surgeon have investigated thoroughly the possible causes for your breast enlargement, and medical therapy has been ruled out as a treatment.

CONSIDERING SURGERY

In gynaecomastia the tissue usually forms just underneath the nipple, and can be on both sides or one side only. True gynaecomastia refers to the enlargement of real breast tissue. With this condition, you would be unable to do anything about the tissue, even through dieting or exercise. Pseudo, or 'false', gynaecomastia refers to the build-up of fatty tissue as a by-product of being overweight.

Gynaecomastia is normally a benign condition, but anyone suffering from breast enlargement should first see their doctor so that they can rule out any other possibilities. In some cases medical therapy can be offered to reduce the gynaecomastia, before surgery is considered. It should be your GP's opinion as much as yours that surgery is required. If they have agreed that surgery is your only option, then the following information should be of use to you.

THE OPERATION

The choice of surgical procedures to reduce male breast tissue is between liposuction, a standard breast reduction operation, or a combination of the two.

DID YOU KNOW?
The history of breast reduction operations began with the treatment of males who had gynaecomastia. Back in the seventh century, Paulus Aegineta, a surgeon in ancient Greece, was the first person to describe the reduction of male breast tissue.

Liposuction Liposuction treatment on its own is reserved for cases where the gynaecomastia is not particularly pronounced and is thought to be primarily due to fat excess. Several small cuts are made either in the armpit or in the breast fold, before a fluid is injected into the area to prepare it for the liposuction. The fat is then sucked out via a cannula. (See pages 118–19 for more details.)

Male breast reduction operation In cases where there is a substantial amount of tissue to be removed, the reduction operation is preferred. There are many ways in which your surgeon can operate, but all of the incisions available will form scars around the dark skin around your nipple, the areola. If the skin is not very saggy, the surgeon will remove the excess breast tissue through an incision below the nipple. Should there be a lot of loose skin the surgeon may have to remove some of it, thus tightening the breast by extending the incision down towards the breast fold. The surgeon then removes the excess skin and tissue and repositions the nipple higher if necessary. Finally, the scars are stitched together.

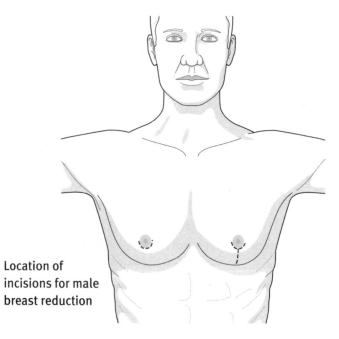

Location of incisions for male breast reduction

THE RECOVERY PROCESS

You will come round from the operation feeling very sore, and you can expect this discomfort to last for the first few days after surgery. Swelling will take a couple of weeks to recede. You are likely to have drainage tubes attached to the operation site, to remove any excess fluid that may gather. You'll be given painkillers as required. You'll need to be able to rest at home for the first couple of days after surgery, and your surgeon will probably advise that you arrange for someone to be with you at all times for the first few days. You'll be instructed to wear a light pressure garment around your chest for a few weeks after surgery, to support the area while it settles.

Most people find that they can go back to work after a week or so, though your surgeon will advise what is best for you – it may be

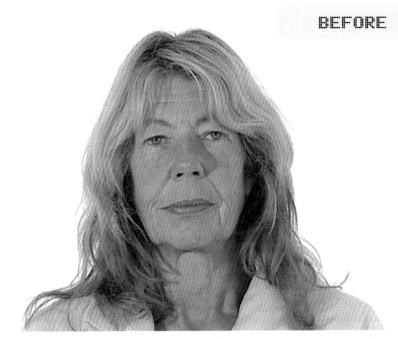

I gave Jackie Ralph a face- and neck lift, blepharoplasty, brow lift and chemical peel, as years of smoking and sunbathing had left her face saggy and drawn.

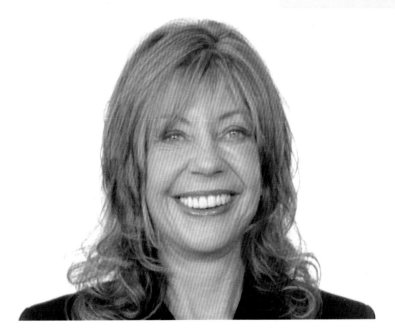

I performed liposuction on Jayne English's thighs and knees, and also gave her a lower blepharoplasty, abdominoplasty (tummy tuck), and a breast augmentation and lift. Jayne had Botox injections too.

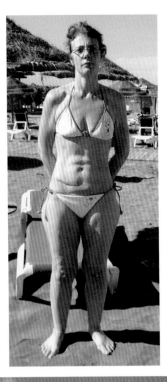

AFTER

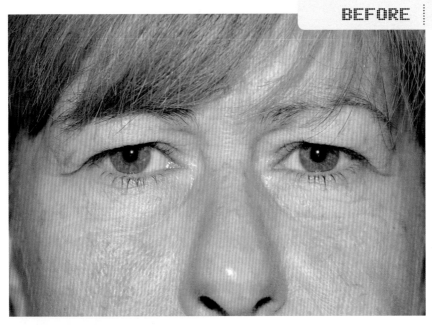

Debbie Ashcroft's endoscopic brow lift and upper and lower blepharoplasty lifted her brows and really brightened her eyes.

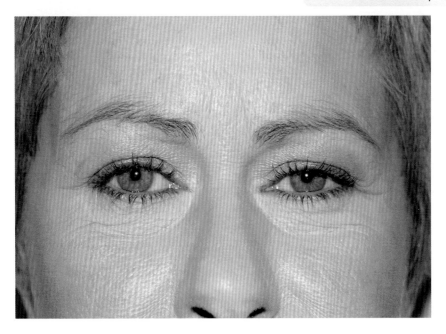

Carole Ward had a full facelift, endoscopic brow lift and blepharoplasty to reduce the jowls and widen her eyes.

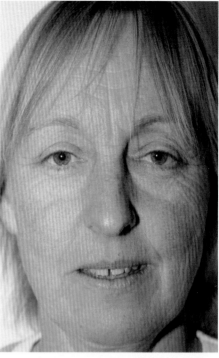

AFTER

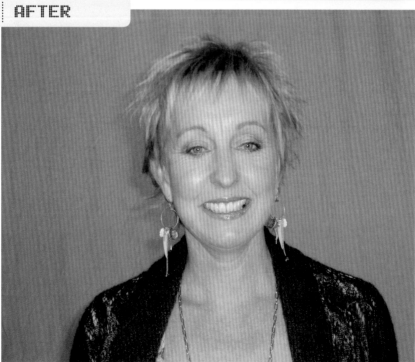

substantially longer. You won't be allowed to drive for at least a week, or to lift any heavy objects or take any exercise for around a month. Your stitches, if you have any, will be removed ten to fourteen days after the procedure. The scars won't completely settle until around a year after the operation. If you notice any signs of infection, for example, hot breasts, pus-like discharge, swelling, pain or fever, contact your surgeon immediately.

DID YOU KNOW?

There may be a chance that you are eligible to have this surgery on the NHS if your doctor deems that treatment is medically necessary. Your GP will be able to find out more once the decision that surgery is an option has been taken.

THE RISKS

Surgery involves a few risks that you should be aware of before opting to have this procedure:

- **Scars** The scars from liposuction are very small and should fade easily, but they will remain on your chest permanently. Depending on the incisions, you may be left with small scars around the nipple or a large anchor-type scar over the breast. Everyone heals differently and so the scars you get will depend on your general health and ability to heal.
- **Loss of sensitivity** You might find that you lose some sensation in your nipple. This is usually temporary, but sometimes can be permanent.
- **Bleeding** This is controlled during surgery but sometimes may continue after the operation, leading to a collection of blood in the breast pocket. This would have to be removed and the bleeding stopped.

- **Infection** You could possibly get an infection after surgery. This is usually treated with antibiotics, which can delay the healing process.
- **Reaction to the anaesthetic** This complication is relevant to all surgery. Your pre-surgery consultation with your anaesthetist should lessen any likelihood of a reaction to the anaesthetic.

IN SHORT

Male breast reduction procedures should only be considered if your GP has been able to rule out a number of other illnesses and has diagnosed gynaecomastia. If your problem is caused by excess weight, you are best advised to try a diet to lose some body fat before you consider surgery. If your condition is true gynaecomastia, then there is a possibility that your operation may be available on the NHS. The surgical techniques are either a simpler version of the female breast reduction operation, or straightforward liposuction. Your surgeon will want to be clear about the diagnosis before proceeding. The operation is carried out under local anaesthetic, but you can expect to feel sore and to be in some pain when you wake up. Sensible aftercare is required to achieve optimal results with this operation. Among the risks associated with the surgery are scarring and loss of sensation, so, as always, proceed with caution. Opt for surgery only when you have researched all of the suitable treatments, have been fully briefed and are completely happy to continue. That said, male breast reduction is a reliable solution for men who are unhappy with the appearance of their chest, and the results can dramatically alter your profile.

FREQUENTLY ASKED QUESTIONS

Q How long does it take?

A Your operation will normally take one and a half to two hours.

Q How long will the results of this operation last?

A The procedures to correct gynaecomastia should have a permanent effect.

Q Will I have to stay in hospital?

A Most surgeons prefer to perform this operation under a light general anaesthetic, so you should be free to leave the same day.

MALE PECTORAL IMPLANTS

Alongside the traditional six-pack that many men aspire to, there are an increasing number of men who wish to have better definition in their chest muscles. Surgical procedures have developed so much that it is now possible for those who want 'pecs' to have implants to enhance them. This is especially useful for body-builders, whose appearance is essential to their profession, and for those who were born with little muscle and for whom no amount of exercise can produce a male-looking chest.

CONSIDERING SURGERY

A pectoral implant operation involves placing silicone implants beneath the pectoral muscle tissue in order to improve the contours of the chest. The implants are made from solid silicone (the same material used for buttock and calf implants). They are usually teardrop-shaped, although other shapes are available, for example with outer convex surface or an inner concave surface. Unlike female breast implants, the fact that pectoral implants are solid means that there is no danger of the implant rupturing. The effect of the surgery is permanent and implants rarely need to be removed as they are designed to last a lifetime.

THE OPERATION

Pectoral implanting is performed via an incision in each armpit.

In the majority of cases, the surgeon will create an incision in the armpit and insert the implant through that incision.

In some cases, however, the surgeon uses an endoscope – a thin tube with a camera attached to the end – to assist with the creation of the pocket so that he does not have to make a large incision. A space between the chest pectoral muscles and the pocket is made so that the implant will fit precisely, with little movement. Having made the pocket, the surgeon ensures that all bleeding is controlled and then inserts the implant through the armpit incision, which is quite difficult because the incision is only about 4cm (1½ inches) long.

Once the implant is in the pocket, it has to be adjusted so that it sits comfortably. During healing, scar tissue will grow around perforations in the implant, ensuring that the implant doesn't move. Usually drains are inserted before the wound is closed, and some sort of strapping helps to immobilize the implants during the early healing period.

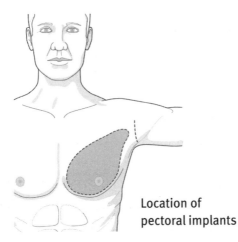

Location of pectoral implants

THE RECOVERY PROCESS

When you wake up, the operation site will be sore and painful. There will be some dressings over the wounds and the chest will be strapped to immobilize the implants. Drains will be placed close to the wound site to relieve any fluid that collects in the area. These may be removed before you leave hospital or may be kept for several days, should there be too much fluid or blood. A nurse will give you instructions about how best to recover. The pain is best described as being like cramp and, although severe at first, will rapidly diminish over a couple of days.

When you get home from hospital, rest as much as you can for a couple of days, making sure you do not lift anything, except for small objects. Most patients find that they can go back to work after around a week. You may take recommended painkillers for any pain, as advised by your surgeon. Take extra care not to raise your blood pressure through exerting yourself for the first few weeks. Any stitches will be removed around a week after the operation. You can expect the pain and tenderness to last for a week and bruising to remain for two weeks. Residual swelling should ease after four or five weeks.

Move your arms with care, but keep your shoulder joints mobile. Do not do any heavy lifting for four weeks after surgery but gradually increase your arm activity. It will be around six weeks before you can exercise again. Contact the surgery if you experience severe pain, bruising, discharge from the wound or fever.

THE RISKS

- **Implant displacement** Very rarely the implant can move if the pectoral muscle moves it during contraction. For this reason it is important that lifting is avoided for four weeks following surgery. Incorrect positioning of the implant can be difficult to correct and will definitely require further surgery.
- **Haematoma/Seroma** (See Glossary)
- **Scars** The scars from this type of implant procedure will be in your armpits. They are made in natural creases and should fade

eventually, although they are permanent and everyone heals (and scars) differently. Talk to your surgeon if you are prone to problem scarring.

- **Infection** This is rare, but if it occurs it is usually treated successfully with antibiotics. If the infection is severe, it may require removal of the implant.
- **Loss of sensation** There is a chance that there will be a difference in skin, nipple and upper arm sensation following a pectoral implant. This is mostly temporary, but it can be permanent.
- **Asymmetry** No one has a symmetrical chest, and sometimes pectoral implants may make this asymmetry noticeable. If it is obvious and distressing it may have to be corrected by changing one of the implants.
- **Reaction to the anaesthetic** This complication is relevant to all surgery. Your pre-surgery consultation with your anaesthetist should lessen any likelihood of a reaction to the anaesthetic.

IN SHORT

Pectoral implants can be used when the chest muscles need to be enhanced in size. The solid silicone implants are placed into the chest via an incision, and the procedure can be assisted endoscopically. The operation is carried out under general anaesthetic, and you can expect to feel sore and to be in some pain for some weeks. Sensible aftercare is required to achieve optimal results. There are few contraindications to having implants, though smokers are at a greater risk of complications and recovery may take longer. Among the risks associated with the surgery are scarring and loss of sensation. So, as always, proceed with caution. Opt for surgery only when you have fully researched all of the suitable treatments, have been fully briefed and are completely happy to continue. Pectoral implants could be a good option if you are unhappy with the appearance of your chest, and the result will thoroughly enhance your chest muscles.

FREQUENTLY ASKED QUESTIONS

Q Will I have to stay in hospital?

A Implants are normally carried out under general anaesthetic, but you should be able to go home the same day.

Q How long does it take?

A Your pectoral implant operation will take between one and two hours to perform.

Q How common is the operation?

A It's not common, though it is increasing in popularity. I have performed twenty of these operations.

Q What can a pectoral implant do?

A A pectoral implant will permanently add bulk behind the pectoral muscle in your chest. The degree of change will depend on the size of implants, and the size of your implants will depend on your build and expectations, which have to be discussed with your surgeon before the operation.

Q What can't it do?

A Pectoral implants will not make you look like Tarzan. Other muscles in the body will have to be exercised so that you remain in proportion. Implants are not available for all body muscles.

Q What are the alternatives?

A It may be that the contours of your chest could be greatly improved by exercise and diet. You could also consider liposuction (page 117), which can be used in body sculpting procedures to add definition in different areas.

THE ARMS

It is one of the first signs that your body is not as young as it used to be: you raise your hand to wave goodbye, and you are confronted with a swinging feeling in your upper arm. Often referred to as 'bat wings', the flabby bits of skin that droop from your upper arms are an inevitable by-product of the tissue's loss of elasticity and the skin's stretching that happen with age.

For most of us, this sagging skin is just a nuisance that we learn to deal with as part of the ageing process, particularly as dieting and some sessions at the gym might help. But for people who have lost a lot of weight and are left with sagging skin that won't be reversed by any amount of exercise, the problem can be severe and unsightly. If this is you, you could consider a surgical procedure called *brachiaplasty*, one of a group of operations that come under the heading of body contouring procedures. Other operations in this group are tummy tucks (page 175), thigh lifts (page 202) and buttock lifts (page 221).

CONSIDERING LOSING WEIGHT? Wait until you have been at your target weight for a while before having this operation in order to get the best permanent results possible.

CONSIDERING SURGERY

One of the things that set these operations apart from other cosmetic surgery procedures is that the scars are usually much worse than you would expect for face or breast operations. This is certainly the case with brachiaplasty. Because there is no natural hiding place for the scar to go, you can expect it to run from your elbow right up to your armpit. But for those who choose this option, the scars are an acceptable consequence of an operation that will give you a better contour.

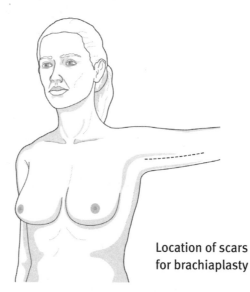

Location of scars
for brachiaplasty

THE OPERATION

An incision is made that runs from your elbow, just inside the lowest point of your arm, up into the armpit. The excess skin is then trimmed away and the wound stitched together again. (Your surgeon will always be conservative in the amount of skin they remove from this area, since the nerves for your arm are close to the site of this operation. If the surgeon were to remove too much skin and pull the remaining skin too tightly, problems with circulation could ensue.) If it is then possible to do so safely, the surgeon may also decide to do some liposuction to the area to rid your arms of any excess fat.

THE RECOVERY PROCESS

You can expect to wake up from this operation with your arms bandaged, and with drains coming from the wounds. These drains are unlikely to be kept in for more than twenty-four hours. You will feel sore and tight, but the discomfort in your arms should get better within a few days. You'll need someone to accompany you home following general anaesthesia, and someone to stay with you for the next day to make sure you can look after yourself. You can take painkillers as directed by your surgeon, if required. Stitches will be removed about one week after your operation. Your surgeon will probably encourage you to stay mobile to prevent clots from forming in your legs.

You can expect to be back at work after around two weeks, but it will be at least four weeks before you can start exercising properly again. Don't be too frightened if at first the scars look red and raised, and bear in mind that scars can take at least a year to mature properly. Contact your surgeon if you notice any signs of infection in the treatment site.

THE RISKS

Arm surgery is a safe procedure. However, some of the reported complications of surgery include the following:

- **Swelling** Your arms will be very swollen after the op. Don't be surprised if the swelling persists for a number of months.
- **Loss of sensation** It is likely that you will experience some loss of sensation in your arms. This is usually temporary. Very occasionally, there can be nerve damage resulting in a permanent loss of sensation.
- **Blood/fluid collection** There is a risk that blood or fluid could collect around the operation site. This is usually a risk monitored during surgery, and any collections are normally drained.

- **Deep vein thrombosis** Your surgeon will monitor you during surgery. Keeping mobile should prevent any clots from forming in the legs after the op.
- **Infection** It is possible that you may get an infection after surgery. This is usually treated with antibiotics, which can delay the healing process.
- **Unfavourable result** Discuss thoroughly with your surgeon beforehand what you hope your surgery will achieve. Be prepared that although your surgeon will make every endeavour to make your arm surgery successful and symmetrical, it cannot be guaranteed.
- **Reaction to the anaesthetic** This complication is relevant to all surgery. Your pre-surgery consultation with your anaesthetist should lessen any likelihood of a reaction to the anaesthetic.

IN SHORT

The brachiaplasty operation to reduce excess skin and fat in the upper arms is one of a number of body contouring procedures that, although fairly new in scope, can offer reliable results and are reasonably safe to undergo. Brachiaplasty cannot make fat arms thin, nor is it a substitute for a healthy diet. It is a corrective measure most often used following severe weight loss but also in cases where the problem is inherited. Any surgeon will want to be satisfied at your consultation that your weight is stable and you have sufficiently lax skin and realistic expectations of what surgery will achieve.

During the operation, your surgeon will make an incision that runs from your elbow right the way along your upper arm into your armpit, before removing any excess fat and skin and closing the wound again. You can expect large and permanent scars after this operation. The risks range from severe bruising and swelling to infection and permanent numbness. Although it will be painful in the immediate post-operative period, you are actively encouraged to get back on your feet fairly speedily following surgery, to prevent clots from forming.

As always proceed with caution. Opt for surgery only when you are sure your weight is stable and you have fully researched and tried other suitable treatments, have been fully briefed and are completely happy to continue. That said, brachiaplasty can be a reliable solution to treat problem residual flab left after weight loss; the results can be dramatic and are usually very successful.

FREQUENTLY ASKED QUESTIONS

Q What can a brachiaplasty do?

A This operation will remove subcutaneous fat and excess skin from your upper arms, sometimes smoothing out the skin in the process.

Q What can't a brachiaplasty do?

A A brachiaplasty cannot make fat arms thin; it can only remove excess skin left after weight loss. It is imperative that you have already reached your intended weight and have maintained that weight for a while before you have this operation. This is because the operation removes only excess skin and subcutaneous fat from a small part of the arm circumference and so it is important that you have as little subcutaneous fat as possible.

Q How long does it take?

A You can expect to be in surgery for at least one to two hours, though it may be considerably longer if you combine the operation with other body contouring procedures, such as a thigh lift or a tummy tuck.

Q Will I have to stay in hospital?

A This operation is normally performed under a general anaesthetic, but you should be able to go home the same day.

Q How long will the results last?

A You can expect your arms to age in the normal way – i.e. a small amount of sagging will occur as the skin becomes lax with age after this procedure, even if you maintain your weight. However, if you gain and lose weight again, you can expect your skin to stretch again, effectively cancelling out the results of your operation.

Q Is there anyone who is not suitable for brachiaplasty?

A If you have stabilized your weight following a diet that has left you with saggy underarm skin, you are reasonably healthy and have good skin, then you are a suitable candidate for this surgery. If, however, you are still losing weight, or your weight tends to fluctuate, you are best advised against this procedure. If you have had a mastectomy, then this operation is not suitable for you. This is because there may be impairment of drainage in lymphatic vessels; this would predispose your arm to swell excessively, which could lead to a serious infection called cellulitis.

Q How common is the operation?

A This is not a very common operation since the procedure is still relatively new in the UK. In 2005, around sixteen thousand brachiaplasty operations were performed in the United States.

Q What are the alternatives?

A There's little else that can be done to remove the kind of excess skin and tissue addressed by a brachiaplasty, since this tissue will not normally respond to exercise or any amount of weight training. However, there may well be a chance that you don't need a full brachiaplasty, and that liposuction (page 115) might achieve the look you are after.

THE STOMACH

For many, the most visible sign that the body is not as young as it once was is a gradual filling out around the waist. For women, this can be exacerbated by the effect that having children has on the stomach muscles. So you decide to do something about it – you do the diet, you start the exercise plan and the pounds begin to fall away. But there is a snag: your skin doesn't fall away with it. And so you end up with an apron of flesh that hangs where your stomach used to be, and no amount of sit-ups will get rid of it. What can you do?

MOTIVATIONS FOR SURGERY

People who undergo this operation generally fall into one of three categories:

- Women who have had children, leaving them with a bulging stomach or hanging flap of skin

- People who have lost a lot of weight

- People who have had previous tummy surgery and want their scars improved

CONSIDERING SURGERY

What you can do is investigate surgery. The operation to flatten and tighten the stomach, called an *abdominoplasty* or *tummy tuck,* is one of the most popular procedures in Britain today. But be warned: this is not a day in the park. The abdominoplasty is one of the most uncomfortable and invasive procedures you can have, so you're probably going to have to get in shape just to cope with it. And you can expect to be left with a hip-to-hip scar as a permanent reminder of how things used to be.

THE LIFE AND TIMES OF A TUMMY

Until you have children, your stomach only has to deal with the bloating effect of menstruation or the occasional extra-large meal. But during pregnancy the muscles of the abdomen are stretched, which can create a permanent weakness of the muscles in the area. Sometimes even a hernia can also occur (when a section of the bowel pokes through the abdomen wall). When your child is born, your stomach should return to a flat position, but whether or not this actually happens depends upon your genes, weight, general health and exercise. For many women, things are never the same again. If the problem is exacerbated by a Caesarean section or further pregnancies, the further you will probably get from your pre-baby belly.

As a woman approaches the menopause, the body starts to store fat around the middle instead of the hips anyway. The already weakened muscles of the stomach inevitably find it difficult to cope, and the belly does one of two things: either it forms an unsightly bulge or it hangs sadly in a flap.

A similar thing can happen to men, though obviously it's less of the babies and more of the overindulging that causes the belly. Since men naturally tend to store their fat around their middle, if they do manage to lose some weight they, too, can be left with saggy skin.

ASSESSING SUITABILITY

Abdominoplasty requires serious aftercare, so before you even book an appointment with a surgeon, consider carefully the long incisions, extended recovery process and emotional rollercoaster you can expect. You need to be fit and healthy to be able to cope with this operation, and your problem has to be sufficiently significant to justify it. There are a number of instances where surgery might not be possible:

- **Weight problem** If you haven't got your weight under control, your surgeon might not want to proceed. This is because if you gain weight after the op, you run the risk of stretching your scars, which could mean that you end up looking worse than before.
- **Deep vein thrombosis or embolism** If you have a history of either of these, the risk of complications in surgery is higher, which may well affect your overall suitability for surgery. Tell your surgeon all about your medical history so they can decide if surgery is an option for you.
- **Diabetes, asthma or any heart problems** If you have a history of any of these, your anaesthetist and surgeon will want to know, to decide if surgery is an option for you.
- **Anaemia** If you are anaemic, then your surgeon will probably recommend that you take iron tablets before the op. There are occasions when loss of blood makes a blood transfusion necessary after a tummy tuck, and anaemia can make this more risky.
- **Blood thinning or clotting problems** If you have any problems with blood thinning or clotting, talk to your surgeon so they can best prepare you for the op.
- **Planning to have a family** If you haven't yet had your family, your surgeon will probably ask you to wait before having surgery.

- **Smoking** Smoking severely impairs your body's ability to heal, and some surgeons will insist that you stop altogether before the operation.

THE IMPORTANCE OF REALISTIC EXPECTATIONS

No one, not even a highly skilled surgeon, can wave a magic wand over you and give you the body of a twenty-year-old. What surgery can do is offer the opportunity to tighten, remove or hoist a little of what is already there. Any potential patient who has unrealistic expectations of surgery will almost certainly be disappointed with the result, regardless of how successful the operation has been, and for this reason, most surgeons will refuse to operate under these circumstances. If, however, you have read and understood what is going to happen, and appreciate that your surgeon will try to achieve the best silhouette possible, then you are more likely to be happy with the outcome.

FIT FOR THE OP: FOUR WAYS TO GET PREPARED FOR SURGERY

Here are some things you can do before the operation that will smooth the way when you come out:

- If you smoke, stop – as soon as you can. You're putting yourself at a far greater risk of post-operative complications and it'll take much longer to get over it.

- In the run-up to surgery, make sure you eat a healthy diet with plenty of fruit and veg to build up your body's capacity to repair itself.

- If you don't do so already, fit some regular exercise into your life in the weeks before the op. A healthier heart and better circulation will benefit you when you have the general anaesthesia.

• Your surgeon will probably tell you to stop taking anything with Vitamin E in it, as well as aspirin, anti-inflammatory drugs or the contraceptive pill, all of which affect the blood's capacity to clot.

TYPES OF ABDOMINOPLASTY

Your surgeon will be able to decide which of the following procedures is best for you. They may suggest any of the following, with or without additional liposuction, in order to obtain the best result:

Standard abdominoplasty The first thing the surgeon does is to inject your stomach with fluid. This is done to reduce bleeding, and, if needed, to prepare the area for any liposuction. Then they will make a large incision that runs from one hip, just above your pubic hairline, over to your other hip. The surgeon also makes an incision around your belly button but leaves it attached to the structures underneath. Once the skin is freed, the surgeon first repairs any hernias present, then separates the skin from the muscle across the whole of your stomach. He then tightens the underlying muscle and trims the excess skin away. Finally, the surgeon makes a hole for your belly button and pulls it through, before stitching the wound site back together. He will leave drains in your stomach to drain away any fluid – these will remain in place for at least twenty-four hours.

Mini abdominoplasty If your stomach doesn't sag too much, then a mini abdominoplasty could be all that you require. With this procedure, the stomach skin is simply pulled down to flatten the contour, and the belly button is left in place. This procedure is suitable for those whose skin is lax only below the tummy button, as it doesn't tighten the skin above the tummy button.

Extended abdominoplasty If the surgeon believes that he can improve the contours of your hip and back with the tummy tuck, he may well recommend an extended abdominoplasty. This requires the incision to be extended on to the hips and towards the back, which allows a greater amount of skin to be hoisted at one time.

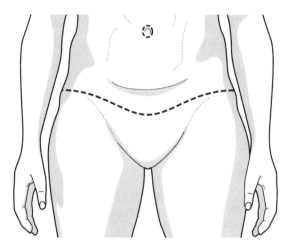

Location of incisions for abdominoplasty

THE RECOVERY PROCESS

This is a major operation, so be prepared for a slow and cumbersome recovery. You'll wake up from the operation feeling very sore and heavily bruised. You'll also feel swollen and your knees will be bent (to reduce pull on the skin and reduce the risk of impaired healing) and on pillows, and two drains will be attached to your stomach. You'll be advised to bend your knees whenever you can, to relieve pressure on your abdomen, and to sleep with your knees bent for the first few days after surgery. You might be wearing compression socks in order to prevent clots from forming. For the first couple of days, you'll be in hospital, where the nursing staff will carefully monitor your progress, as you are at greatest risk of complications during this time. The drains will probably be removed just before you leave hospital.

Once you get home, you'll be given painkilling medication and advised to get mobile pretty quickly, though you need to take care not to stretch or strain too much. Recovery can be a slow and emotionally draining process. Stitches will be removed around ten days after surgery, and you'll be advised to wear a pressure garment after this to ease the swelling in the first few weeks. Most people find that they can go back to work two to four weeks after surgery. Driving is usually possible within two weeks, but it'll be at least four to six weeks before you can return to all normal activities, such as exercising.

It can take up to six months for the swelling to go down and up to a year for the scars to mature, so although you'll probably feel flatter fairly quickly, the results of your op can't really be judged for a while. How you heal will also depend on how healthy you were before the op too.

Finally, do not hesitate to contact your surgeon if you notice any signs of infection or have a high temperature, bleeding, wound separation, a pus-like discharge or heavy pain.

GETTING THE RIGHT SUPPORT It is important that you enlist the support of someone who is sensible and isn't squeamish to look after you in the immediate post-operation period. This is not always the person closest to you, and you should think carefully about who has the time and patience to help. They must be able to change dressings, help you wash, perhaps even remove the drains in your stomach. It can be an unsightly business, but you need to be able to concentrate on yourself after the op and not have to worry about anyone else. If you have a family, think about the environment you need to recover best in. You'll be back on the school run much quicker if you have had a good rest after the op, and this is not always possible at the family home.

THE RISKS

As you know by now, this is a major op. You should be aware of the following possible complications, though most of them are highly unlikely:

- **Bleeding** The risk of bleeding is highest immediately after the operation and is usually treated straight away with no long-term effects. The risk is higher in men than in women.
- **Infection** It is rare for a major infection to occur but if one does, it can usually be treated easily with no long-term effects. You are also at a greater risk of chest infection after an abdominoplasty.
- **Poor scarring** Talk to your surgeon if you heal badly. Smokers are at a greater risk of bad scarring.
- **Haematoma/Seroma** (See Glossary)
- **Loss of sensation** Most people lose some sensation between the belly button and the pubic hairline after the operation. It should return in time as the nerves repair themselves, but occasionally it can be permanent. There have also been occasions when patients have been left with a permanent tingling sensation either across the stomach or at the top of the leg.
- **Tissue problems** Sometimes the fat in your abdomen can die as a result of the operation, resulting in lumpiness.
- **Necrosis** (See Glossary)
- **Reaction to the anaesthetic** This complication is relevant to all surgery. Your pre-surgery consultation with your anaesthetist should lessen any likelihood of a reaction to the anaesthetic.

IN SHORT

The tummy tuck operation to reduce excess skin and fat from the abdomen is one of a number of body contouring procedures that can offer reliable and dramatic results. However, abdominoplasty cannot make you thin, nor is it a substitute for a healthy diet. It is a corrective measure most often used following severe weight loss or multiple pregnancies. Any surgeon will want to be satisfied at your consultation that your weight is stable, you are fit and healthy, you have sufficiently lax skin and your expectations of what surgery will achieve are realistic. They may also require you to prepare for surgery through an exercise routine or further weight loss.

During the operation, your surgeon will make an incision that runs from hip to hip, remove the excess skin and close the wound. He will also move your belly button to a higher position. You can expect large and permanent scars after this operation. The risks associated with this procedure range from infection and swelling to permanent loss of sensation. Extensive aftercare is required and you will experience a prolonged period of discomfort. That said, you are actively encouraged to get mobile and back on your feet fairly speedily following surgery to prevent any clots from forming in your blood.

As always, proceed with caution. Opt for surgery only when you are sure your weight is stable and you have fully researched and tried other suitable treatments, have been fully briefed and are completely happy to continue. In general, the tummy tuck can be a reliable solution to treat problem residual flab left after pregnancy or weight loss, and the results can be dramatic and are usually very successful.

FREQUENTLY ASKED QUESTIONS

Q How long has the operation been around?
A Surgeons have been refining the technique to flatten the stomach since the turn of the twentieth century.

Q How common is the operation?
A This is a common operation as the results are reliable and

often dramatic. In the United States in 2005, nearly 170,000 abdominoplasty procedures were carried out. I perform this surgery at least three times a month, and I have noticed a steady increase in women wanting the operation.

Q Is it painful?

A Generally surgeons agree that the abdominoplasty is one of the most uncomfortable operations in cosmetic surgery.

Q How long does the operation take?

A The amount of time can vary according to whether or not you have liposuction and any other procedures, but the abdominoplasty itself takes around two hours.

Q Will I have to stay in hospital?

A Abdominoplasty is carried out under general anaesthesia, so you'll be in hospital for at least one, and probably two, nights.

Q What can a tummy tuck do?

A A tummy tuck will remove the excess skin in your abdomen, tighten the muscles underneath, while at the same time flattening its appearance.

Q What can't a tummy tuck do?

A Abdominoplasty does not make fat people thin, nor can it give you back a pre-pregnancy completely flat stomach.

Q How long do the results last?

A If you don't gain any weight after the op, you can say goodbye to a flabby tummy for ever. However, your skin will continue to age in the normal way, losing elasticity with the passing years.

Q What are the alternatives?

A If your problem is a flap of skin that is resistant to exercise, the only way to rid yourself of it is with surgery. However, if your problem is mild sagging or a pot belly, it may be that this can be addressed just by liposuction (page 115).

REMEMBER The tummy tuck operation should not be seen as an alternative to diet and exercise and it should never be undertaken without a serious effort to lose excess fat first. Your surgeon will want to know what you have done to improve the area yourself before any operation. In any case, you could find that regular trips to the gym might provide all the lift you need without having to resort to the pain that comes with the scalpel.

THE TUMMY BUTTON

Your tummy button is essentially a scar from your umbilical cord, which was cut away when you were born. What it looks like depends upon how well you heal and the strength of your abdominal muscles; therefore no two are the same. The *umbilicoplasty* operation tries to improve the look of your tummy button, whatever the aesthetic problem might be.

Tummy buttons basically fall into two categories: either the scar has pulled into the abdomen (nicknamed an 'innie') or the scar protrudes from the abdomen (an 'outie'). Since fashion seems to have a preference for the innie version, cosmetic surgeons have developed the umbilicoplasty operation in response. It is usual for this procedure to be combined with a tummy tuck, though it can be performed on its own.

CONSIDERING SURGERY

There are a number of reasons why you might be unhappy with your tummy button. Some babies are born with small hernias, or you might develop one later in life – these are small sections of the intestine that protrude through the muscle wall. They can protrude next to the tummy button, and are corrected by this surgery. But perhaps your tummy button is just too small or too big, too long or too flat, lopsided or completely hidden, or it sticks out too much, all of which might see you heading for the surgeon's office.

DID YOU KNOW?
Your tummy button is not determined by genetics in any way. It is a scar that is created at birth. Even the tummy buttons of identical twins differ, providing a useful way of telling them apart early on!

THE OPERATION

Your surgeon will make incisions inside your tummy button in order to be able to manipulate it. This may involve the removal of some tissue, correcting a scar or repairing a hernia. If the surgeon removes any skin, he will repair the wound with stitches, which are normally dissolvable. Any scars should be hidden within the tummy button after surgery.

THE RECOVERY PROCESS

You can expect to be back on your feet within a day since this operation is simple and complications are rare. You'll come round from the op probably feeling a bit sore and the area will be tender to touch, but any pain you get should be easily controlled with painkillers. Your tummy button will probably be covered with a dressing that can be removed once your doctor has given the all-clear. However, if you do notice any signs of infection, do not hesitate to contact your surgeon.

THE RISKS

You can expect some bruising and swelling which can take a week or so to recede. Other risks are those associated with all surgery, such as infection, blood or fluid collection, numbness or a reaction to the anaesthetic. These complications are very unlikely following umbilicoplasty as the operation is not particularly invasive, but make sure you talk these through with your surgeon beforehand so that you are fully prepared. There will, of course, be a scar from the surgery, but it should be well hidden.

FREQUENTLY ASKED QUESTIONS

Q How long will the results of the operation last?

A As long as you maintain your weight and do not have further pregnancies, the results of this operation should be permanent.

Q Is there anyone who is unsuitable for tummy button surgery?

A If you have realistic expectations and are in good general health, you should be a good candidate for surgery. If you are prone to problem scarring, talk to your surgeon before the op so that he can adapt his incisions to offer the neatest result in your case.

Q How long does it take?

A You'll be in surgery for about an hour.

Q Will I have to stay in hospital?

A This operation is normally performed using a local anaesthetic, so you will be awake during it, but you will be drowsy. You'll almost certainly be able to return home that day.

Q What can't umbilicoplasty do?

A It will not make your stomach flat. If this is the result you are after, talk to your surgeon about abdominoplasty (page 175), though that is a far more extensive and demanding operation.

THE PENIS

Everyone has insecurities about their body, whether it's their jowls, saggy arms or knobbly feet. Many males have an insecurity about their penis, even though penises really do come in all shapes and sizes. And unfortunately, since the penis is not a muscle, no amount of trips to the gym are going to affect its size. For most, this insecurity will pass, but for some it can be the cause of quite severe psychological distress.

CONSIDERING SURGERY

The first thing you should do if you are seriously considering opting for a procedure is talk to a professional such as a counsellor or relationship therapist, who can help you understand your concerns and discuss your motivations for surgery. It may be that your worries can be resolved without the need for theatre. In fact, there are surgeons who insist that anyone considering penis augmentation surgery undergo counselling before a procedure.

Although the field of penis augmentation surgery, or *phalloplasty*, is relatively well established, the results are controversial. There are currently no reliable statistics relating to the long-term effects of operations in this field, and so you should proceed with extra care. I do not perform this kind of surgery within my practice, though there are a number of surgeons in the UK who do. However, it may take some time to find a suitably experienced surgeon in the field. The view of a large number of experts remains that for anything other than corrective or reconstructive surgery, it is difficult to merit a procedure. This is not to say that it won't in the future, of course, but at the present time this field is still considered experimental rather than standard procedure.

There are nevertheless surgical procedures you can consider that are designed to increase the size of your penis. Either the length can be augmented or the girth can be increased, or both can be augmented at the same time.

HOW LONG HAVE THESE PROCEDURES BEEN IN USE? The history of penile augmentation is relatively short. Corrective surgery to treat severe shortening due to congenital abnormalities (from birth), post-surgery (for cancer or Peyronie's disease) or trauma (amputation) has been offered since the seventies. The United States was the first to offer cosmetic lengthening and widening in the eighties. The procedure utilizing liposuction and fat injection has been available as a treatment for increasing girth since 1991.

INCREASING PENIS LENGTH

The technique that most surgeons use to increase the length of the penis is to sever the suspensory ligament that attaches the penis to the pubic bone. Once this is cut, the penis, which was lying under the pubic bone, drops and more of it is exposed, giving the illusion of increased length. The skin on the penis will generally accommodate this increase in length, though there are occasions where a skin graft might be required. The surgeon will make a 2.5cm (1 inch) V-shaped incision in the pubic-hair region, from where they will locate the ligament and cut it. There is no scar on the penis itself. The ligament is then reattached lower down on the pubic bone.

Some surgeons recommend the use of penile weights to further enhance length following this procedure.

Whether or not you will see any increase in the length of your penis is debatable. Reports of up to a 50 per cent increase have been cited, but results of these operations have never been systematically tested and so it is impossible to say what is actually the case. It is true to say that some patients experience no lengthening at all after this operation, while others detect a definite increase. I would advise that you talk to your surgeon about the results they have achieved in their patients and ask for photographic evidence.

INCREASING PENIS WIDTH

Fat injection There is a technique by which surgeons can increase the girth of the penis with liposuction and fat transfer. Fat is normally removed from the tummy using a metal cannula (hollow tube), and then injected into the shaft of the penis. This injection temporarily makes the penis wider, but as the fat is slowly absorbed by the body, any gain is eventually lost. Repeat injections are usually required and so you should ask your surgeon how much of the fat injected is likely to survive permanently. Apart from the fact that this is only a temporary measure, injecting fat into the penis is an unpredictable and inexact science. Irregularities of the penis are commonplace after this procedure, and while the fat is present your erection will be much softer than before.

Dermal fat grafts An alternative method that some surgeons have used involves taking a graft of your dermis (the layer of skin and tissue under your outermost layer of skin) from somewhere else on your body, or a human cadaver graft that has been extensively tested and prepared for use. This is inserted via a small incision into the shaft of the penis and wrapped around the shaft, until the desired thickness is reached. In theory, this technique can offer better results than injecting fat into the base of the penis. However, what you gain in uniformity, you could possibly lose in sensation. The procedure is more involved than fat injections, and so the risk of complications is inevitably higher. To date, there has been no reliable testing of this procedure, and so no long-term results exist.

THE RECOVERY PROCESS

Although these operations involve minor incisions and are relatively quick, you can expect some discomfort in the post-operative period due to the sensitive nature of the operation site. You can expect to wake up from the operation with some swelling, and you will feel sore. During the first couple of weeks, you need to be extra-vigilant about personal hygiene to prevent infection. You will probably need a week off work to rest. Unless dissolvable stitches were used, your sutures will need to be removed after around ten days. It'll be a month before you can exercise or go swimming, and at least six weeks before you can recommence sexual activity.

> **DID YOU KNOW?**
> Between 1998 and 2005, surgeons conducting a study in this field talked to nearly fifty men who underwent augmentation operations. The average increase in size was around 12mm ($^1/_2$ inch) but two thirds said they were unhappy with the results.

THE RISKS

Some may argue that when it comes to the penis, any threat of complications is too big a risk, but if you are seriously considering one of these operations, be aware of the following:

- **Loss of sensation** Sensation in your penis may be affected.

- **Impotence** There have been reports of impotence following the procedure, though this is extremely rare.
- **Effect on erection** Cutting the suspensory ligament can affect your erection. It may be a bit wobbly, or start lower down, or stick down or out instead of up. However, this shouldn't necessarily interfere with intercourse. Fat injection will cause it to feel softer. Any increase in size, if there is one, will not necessarily translate into an increase in size when erect.
- **Pubic hair growth** With lengthening, you may find that pubic hair grows on the top of your penis, which might require shaving.
- **Necrosis** If skin was grafted on to your penis to accommodate the length created, this skin may die as it becomes affected by a reduced blood supply.
- **Deformed appearance** A fat injection may cause your penis to develop nodules of fat on it, as fat does not settle in a uniform pattern; this can make it look deformed. After lengthening, your penis may seem to extend from your scrotum, not your abdomen. Also, there are no guarantees that fat injection will increase your girth in a regular fashion.

IN SHORT

There are surgical procedures available to enhance the size of the penis, though they are yet to be subject to large-scale reliability testing, and so patients are advised to proceed with caution and take time to find the right surgeon for the procedure. Any surgeon will want to be clear about your motivations before proceeding, and be sure that your expectations of what surgery can achieve are realistic. If you are still intent on the operation, you can increase penis size by length and/or girth. To increase the length, surgeons cut the ligament that pulls the penis into the abdomen, so that the penis drops, offering an illusion of extra length. To increase girth, your choice is between fat injections, which have unpredictable results, and fat grafting. Grafting is probably more reliable, but it runs the risk of affecting sensation in the penis. The operation is usually carried out under general anaesthetic, and you can expect to be in some pain for a time after the op. You will have to take extra care with regular washing to avoid infection of the wounds in the recovery period. As always, opt for surgery only when you have fully researched all of the suitable treatments, understand the associated risks and complications, have been fully briefed and are completely happy to continue.

FREQUENTLY ASKED QUESTIONS

Q How long does it take?

A This surgery will take around an hour to perform, possibly longer if you decide to have both lengthening and widening done at the same time.

Q Will I need to stay in hospital?

A If you do opt for surgery, you're likely to have it done under a general anaesthetic, but you will probably be able to leave that day.

Q What are the alternatives?

A There are a number of non-surgical alternatives available, though, to date, none has been proven to work on a long-term basis, so consider all with a healthy dose of scepticism. Examples of non-surgical treatments include vacuum pumps, penile weights and hormone therapy. Since obesity can make the penis appear smaller, you might find that a healthy diet, some regular exercise and losing a few pounds produces a perceptible improvement. Shaving some of your pubic hair can add to the illusion of extra length.

THE VAGINA

Both childbirth and the menopause can permanently alter the
size and elasticity of the vagina, impacting on sex life. In the past,
women accepted this as a natural consequence of having a family
or getting older, but in recent years surgeons have developed a
number of techniques that can tighten the vagina to restore it to
a pre-baby size, or to remove the clitoral hood in order to improve
sensation during sexual intercourse. These are not necessarily
operations limited to women who have completed their families, as
some women seek this operation because they are unhappy with
the natural size of their vagina anyway, and wish to take action to
improve their sex life. More recently, surgeons have developed an
operation in response to the growing number of women who are
unhappy with the size, shape or appearance of their labia. Both of
these operations are relatively straightforward, and the results are
a reliable way of improving both aesthetics and sensation. However,
these operations will not improve your situation if your problem
is incontinence or poor pelvic floor muscles. These are urological
conditions that you should contact your GP about.

If you are one of the many women who are considering this surgery,
you may have some difficulty finding an experienced practitioner in
the UK, since it is not very common at the moment. Though it is not
a surgical operation that I perform, this chapter should give you an
idea of the procedures available.

ABOUT THE VAGINA

The vagina is the muscular tube that connects the vulva (external female genitals) on the outside of your body to the cervix of the uterus on the inside. The vulva and the urethra opening to the bladder are covered by two folds of fleshy tissue. The outer fold is called the labia majora, and the inner fold the labia minora. The clitoris is at the front of the vulva (which is the collective name for the labia, clitoris, vaginal opening and urethra). In general, the outer labia are larger than the inner labia. However, as women come in all shapes and sizes, this may well not be the case. *Vaginoplasty* is the procedure to alter the size of the vagina, while *labiaplasty* alters the size and shape of the labia.

When a woman gives birth, her vagina expands to between two and three times its normal size. Though it is designed to stretch, for many the vagina never recovers fully to its pre-baby size. In addition, a woman can also sustain various other injuries when she has a baby, ranging from incidental tearing to an episiotomy incision. In fact, more than eight out of every ten women experience some kind of internal injury during childbirth. Of these, at least 60 per cent need stitches. It is unsurprising, therefore, that the process of childbirth generally leaves women with a weakened and slackened vagina. This often impacts on sensation, both for the woman and her partner.

CONSIDERING SURGERY

If you book a consultation for this surgery, you can expect to have a frank and open discussion about your motivations and possibly your sex life. These are uncommon operations in an intimate area, and your surgeon will want to be clear that you have a valid reason for opting for surgery, that you actually require it and that you have realistic expectations of what surgery can achieve. The surgeon might well suggest that you visit a counsellor or therapist as part of this process. The surgeon will also need to examine you as part of your consultation. You may wish to bring along a friend for support, who can remain in the room while this happens, or you can always ask a practice nurse to be present during this time.

TYPES OF SURGERY

Vaginoplasty This is an umbrella term for the standard gynaecological operations that correct structural defects in the vagina. There are many types of surgery, but the most common involves tightening the muscles so as to narrow the vagina, in order to repair any internal damage caused by childbirth or to improve sensation during sexual intercourse. Your surgeon removes a slim section of the vagina and stitches together the remaining sections. This reduces the amount of vaginal lining and therefore tightens the muscles. Any scarring is present only inside the vagina.

Labiaplasty This is an operation to trim and reshape the folds of the labia, as some people consider that shorter and smaller labia constitute a more youthful contour. This is done by simply trimming any excess tissue away along the desired shape and stitching the wound; any scars, though present along the labia themselves, should eventually fade. Some surgeons prefer to remove a wedge-shaped section of the labia at the back, which leaves virtually undetectable scars. Both procedures can be done using a laser or a scalpel.

Clitoral hoodectomy Also called clitoral circumcision or *clitoridotomy*, this is an operation to remove, reduce or split the skin surrounding the clitoris to improve sensitivity. It can be offered to women as an operation that may improve sex life through improving sensation in the clitoris, thus in theory making it quicker for a woman to reach orgasm. The surgeon simply excises the tissue that forms the clitoral hood to leave the clitoris exposed.

Hymen reconstruction In this operation, which is often done for cultural reasons, the surgeon simply stitches together the remaining hymen after it has been broken by sexual intercourse, exercise or the use of tampons.

Liposuction It is possible to have the fat of the pubic mound removed with liposuction, therefore reducing its size. This can be done either on its own or in conjunction with liposuction on the thighs or tummy.

Fat injections Your surgeon might recommend a fat injection to plump out the pubic mound or the labia majora.

Laser therapy There have been reports of lasers being used in the treatment of labial wrinkles.

Hair transplantation There is a possibility that your surgeon could add hair to the pubic mound.

THE RECOVERY PROCESS

You can expect to feel sore and swollen after these procedures, and you can expect some pain at first. You might experience some light bleeding for the first twenty-four hours, but you should have full sensation and normal function in the area. You will need someone to accompany you home after the operation if you had a general anaesthetic and look after you for at least twenty-four hours. You'll be off work for around a week, so take it easy for a few days and remember to be vigilant about your personal hygiene during this time to prevent the likelihood of any infection. You can shower again after a couple of days, and you should feel back to normal in about ten days. Avoid using tampons or constricting underwear, horse riding or cycling for about three weeks. It will take about six weeks for the area to completely heal. Most women are advised to wait this long before resuming penetrative sex.

THE RISKS

All surgery carries risks, but these procedures are generally considered very safe. Nonetheless, be aware of the following possible complications:

- **Overcorrection** Sometimes the surgeon may remove too much tissue, which can make the vagina too small for penetrative sex to be comfortable. However, the scar normally stretches over time, and so the problem sorts itself out.
- **Infection** Occasionally patients can be prone to urinary infections as the bacteria normally around the anus can be pulled closer to the vagina. Vigilant personal hygiene should prevent this.
- **Unfavourable result** It may be that after surgery you are disappointed with the result, particularly if the scarring is bad. You need to have realistic expectations that this surgery is not an exact science and appreciate that everyone heals differently.
- **Bleeding** This is controlled during surgery but some bleeding may continue after the operation, occasionally with blood collecting. This collected blood may need to be removed.
- **Altered sensation** It is possible that sensation can be altered by surgery.
- **Perforation of the bowel** This is a serious complication that could occur through human error, though it is very rare indeed.

IN SHORT

Surgical procedures are available to enhance the shape and size of your vagina, labia and pubic mound, though these operations are still fairly new in the UK, and so patients may find it hard to find a suitable surgeon. Any surgeon will want to be clear about your motivations and expectations before proceeding. A surgeon can alter the shape and size of your vagina by removing a section of the tissue inside and stitching the remainder back together. The operation to alter the labia is also very straightforward, since the surgeon is able to easily trim the labia to suit. Other surgical procedures that can be used include liposuction or fat injections to alter the contours of the area, stitching together a broken hymen and laser therapy to improve wrinkles. Whether you stay in hospital depends on the operation you have, but most procedures shouldn't take more than an hour and all are easy to recover from. You will have to take extra care with regular washing to avoid infection to the wounds in the recovery period. As always, opt for surgery only when you have fully researched all of the suitable treatments, understand the associated risks and complications, have been fully briefed and are completely happy to continue.

FREQUENTLY ASKED QUESTIONS

Q Will I need to stay in hospital?
A This largely depends on who is performing your operation and what is being done. The most likely scenario is that you will be put under general anaesthetic and required to stay in overnight, although there have been reports of labiaplasty being performed using an epidural so that patients can tell the surgeon during the op how they want to look.

Q How long will the results last?
A Although you may experience some natural slackening with age, the results of these operations should be permanent.

Ⓠ What are the alternatives?

Ⓐ Apart from learning to live with what nature and your life have given you, you could try pelvic floor exercises. These can boost vaginal tightness, which may in turn restore some previously lost sensation.

THE THIGHS

Whether it's caused by cellulite or just an inherited pear shape, few women are truly happy with their thighs. That said, there are a number of things that can be done to make them look better. A simple diet might reduce the size and therefore do the trick; or if it's localized fat deposits that trouble you, there's always liposuction (page 115) to investigate. That is, unless you become overweight. In overweight people the skin in the legs is stretched. In severe obesity, more skin is actually created, too. If you then successfully lose the weight, what you are likely to be left with is wrinkly and sagging loose skin where your fat used to be. This skin is unsightly and unforgiving, and is completely unresponsive to exercise. So what can you do about it?

CONSIDERING SURGERY

There is a procedure that can remove the excess skin and redrape what is left so that you can say goodbye to the loose skin that hangs from your thighs. It's called a thigh lift, or *thighplasty*, and is one of a number of body-contouring procedures for use with patients who have achieved dramatic weight loss. Other examples are the tummy tuck (page 175), buttock lift (page 221) and arm lift (page 169). These procedures are frequently carried out in combination to enhance the overall effect of surgery.

When a thigh lift is combined with a buttock lift, it is called a lower body lift. If you are considering a lower body lift, the information found here and in the buttock lift chapter (page 221) will provide you with most of what you need to know. With a lower body lift, you'll be under general anaesthetic for longer, and it'll take longer to get back on your feet, too.

Like a tummy tuck, a thigh lift is not for the faint-hearted. This is one of the most painful and invasive procedures you can elect to have. You need to be fit and healthy to undergo this operation, so you will probably have to get in shape just to cope with it. If you do opt for surgery, you can expect to be left with a lengthy scar as a permanent reminder of how things used to be. In addition, a thigh lift requires serious aftercare, particularly as it is one of the operations most prone to infection. So before you even book an appointment with a surgeon, consider carefully the long incisions, extended recovery process and emotional rollercoaster involved.

At your consultation, your surgeon will examine your thighs to make sure that there is enough loose skin to merit the procedure. He may also want to take measurements and, with your permission, take photographs of your thighs to provide material for a before-and-after comparison. (For more advice about the consultation process see pages 331–2.)

THE OPERATION

The surgeon will make incisions extending from the inside of your groin around and on to your buttocks. He will then remove the excess fat and skin by cutting elliptical segments. The skin that is left over is pulled smooth and stitched back together. The incisions are designed to be hidden underneath a bikini. If there is a large amount of excess skin on the inner thigh, the surgeon may also make a vertical incision stretching down towards your knee; this allows for the skin to be pulled tighter in a horizontal direction as well as the lift up. In either case, you can expect to be left with a long scar. If both the front and the outer thigh are affected by loose skin, the surgeon may have to extend the incision all the way round the thigh and tighten the whole circumference of the thigh. This is called a full thigh lift.

PERSONAL HYGIENE IS IMPORTANT The position of the incisions used in the thigh lift operation put you at a higher risk of infection than normal. If an infection occurs it will lengthen your recovery time and it could mean that the scars you are left with are worse than expected. This is why it is vitally important that you maintain a high standard of personal hygiene following this surgery. Most surgeons will advise that you wash with unperfumed soap and water following every trip to the toilet.

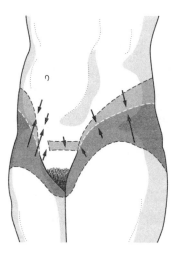

The thigh lift operation

THE RECOVERY PROCESS

This is a major operation, so be prepared for a slow and cumbersome recovery that involves a moderate to high amount of pain. You'll wake up from the operation feeling very sore and swollen. You may feel sick and be unable to go to the toilet at first. You'll also feel bruised, probably all down your legs, and you'll have drains coming from the operation site to drain any excess fluid after surgery. (The drains will probably be removed just before you leave hospital.) You'll probably be wearing a compression garment in order to prevent clots from forming inside the wound. For the first couple of days, you'll be in hospital, where the nursing staff will carefully monitor your progress, as you are at greatest risk of complications during this time.

Once you get home, it is important to have created a good environment for your recovery. You'll be given painkilling medication and advised to get mobile pretty quickly, though you need to take care not to stretch or strain too much. Stitches will be removed around ten days after surgery, and you'll be advised to wear a pressure garment after this, to ease the swelling in the first few weeks. Most people find that they can go back to work two or three weeks after surgery, but it'll be at least four to six weeks before you can return to all normal activities, such as exercising or driving.

It can take up to six months for the swelling to go down and up to a year for the scars to mature, so the results of your op can't really be judged for a while. The operation site will probably be numb, and this can take months to return to normal. How you heal will depend on how healthy you were before the op. Finally, do not hesitate to contact your surgeon if you notice any signs of infection or have a high temperature, bleeding, wound separation, pus-like discharge or intense pain.

THE RISKS

As you know by now, this is a major op. You should be aware of the following possible complications, though most of them are highly unlikely:

- **Infection** Since this operation involves the groin, you are at an increased risk of infection if you do not keep the area clean after every bowel movement.
- **Bleeding** The risk of bleeding is highest immediately after the operation and is usually treated straight away with no long-term effects. The risk is higher in men than in women.
- **Poor scarring** Talk to your surgeon if you heal badly. Smokers are at a greater risk of bad scarring.
- **Haematoma/Seroma** (See Glossary)
- **Loss of sensation** Most people lose some sensation between the pubic hairline and the knee after the operation. It should return in time as the nerves repair themselves, but occasionally it can be permanent. There have also been reports of patients who have been left with a permanent tingling sensation in the area.
- **Injury to the lymphatic system** If this occurs during surgery, you can expect to experience a large amount of swelling for a number of weeks. The problem usually corrects itself in time.
- **Reaction to the anaesthetic** This complication is relevant to all surgery. Your pre-surgery consultation with your anaesthetist should lessen any likelihood of a reaction to the anaesthetic.

IN SHORT

The thigh lift operation to reduce excess skin and fat from the thighs is one of a number of body contouring procedures that can offer reliable and dramatic results. However, this operation alone cannot make your thighs slim, nor is it a substitute for a healthy diet. It is a corrective measure most often used following severe weight loss. Any surgeon will want to be satisfied at your consultation that your weight is stable, you are fit and healthy, you have sufficiently lax skin and your expectations of what surgery will achieve are realistic.

During the operation, the surgeon will make an incision that runs from the groin round to the top of the buttock. They will remove excess skin, lift and tighten what is left and close the wound. The risks associated with this procedure range from infection to permanent loss of sensation. Extensive aftercare is required. However, you are actively encouraged to get back on your feet fairly speedily. As always, proceed with caution. Opt for surgery only when you are sure your weight is stable and you have fully researched and tried other suitable treatments that might be available to you, you have been fully briefed and are completely happy to continue. For many, a thigh lift could be a reliable solution to treat problem residual skin left after dramatic weight loss, and is normally very successful.

FREQUENTLY ASKED QUESTIONS

Q How common is the operation?

A Since the thigh lift is normally only performed in cases of extreme weight loss, it is still uncommon in Britain, though over 12,000 were performed in the United States in 2005. I have performed this operation around fifty times.

Q How long do the effects of this operation last?

A The effect of a thigh lift should be permanent. However, if you gain weight again after your surgery, you can expect your skin to once again stretch, and so the effect of the surgery will be lost. As ever, the ageing process will continue and the skin will gradually become more lax.

Q How long does this operation take?

A A thigh lift normally takes around three to four hours.

Q Will I have to stay in hospital?

A The operation is performed with a general anaesthetic, so you can expect to be in hospital for at least one night, in fact, probably two.

Q What can a thigh lift do?

A A thigh lift can remove excess skin from your thighs, lift and tighten the skin in the area and perhaps slightly slim the circumference of your thighs.

Q What can't a thigh lift do?

A This operation cannot make fat thighs thin, nor can it get rid of chubby knees or saggy buttocks. If this is you, it may be that liposuction is the treatment you should consider.

Q Is there anyone who is not suitable for a thigh lift?

A If you are still losing weight, then wait. Your surgery will have a better chance of success if your weight has been stable for a while and you are within a healthy weight range. If you have any problems with your legs, such as varicose veins, inflamed blood vessels or poor circulation, you should talk these through with your surgeon as it may well affect your suitability for surgery.

Q What are the alternatives?

A If the thought of such drastic surgery fills you with fear, there is now the possibility that a similar effect to surgery can be gained using the thread lift technique (page 275), though the efficacy of this treatment is still a matter of discussion. If your sagging isn't particularly extensive, it could be that liposuction alone (page 115) might provide the lift you require without the need for a lengthy recovery and long scars. Your surgeon will advise you.

THE CALVES

Although still fairly uncommon at the moment, an operation has been developed in response to the increasing number of people who wish to have better definition in their leg calf muscles. It is carried out by inserting special silicone implants under the lining of the calf muscles. This is an operation that may be especially useful for body-builders, who desire large muscles with better definition, and for those who were born with little calf muscle which no amount of exercise will change.

DID YOU KNOW?
The part of the leg that runs from the knee to the ankle is called the cnemis.

THE OPERATION

The calf implant operation involves placing a solid silicone implant beneath the muscle tissue envelope in order to improve the contour of your leg. Unlike female breast implants, there is no gel inside the implant, which means that there is no danger of the implant rupturing. The effect of the surgery is permanent; the implants rarely need to be removed as they are designed to last a lifetime, and complications only very rarely occur.

The surgeon will make an incision in the crease at the back of your knee before creating a pocket for the implant in the back of the leg. They then place the implant on top of the leg muscle, between the muscle and its fibrous envelope. Sometimes two implants of different sizes and shapes are used if the whole calf muscle is undeveloped. The implant is held in place by the pocket made in the fibrous tissue surrounding the muscle and by perforations in the implant that allow the fibrous tissue to grow through. Drains may be left to drain the wounds, and the incision is closed with sutures.

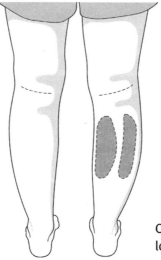

Calf implant
locations

THE RECOVERY PROCESS

When you wake up from the operation, your legs will be painful and will be bandaged. You can expect the pain, swelling, tenderness and bruising to remain for the first few days, but you may take recommended painkillers, as advised by your surgeon. When you get home from hospital, rest for a couple of days with your legs elevated, gradually increasing your walking. Aim to get mobile fairly quickly, to prevent any clots from forming, and remember when resting always to elevate your feet, at least for the first week. It may be difficult to walk for two to three days or more, and it is best to get about using crutches (supplied by the clinic) to relieve any stretching of the calf muscles. Do not do any heavy lifting for a couple for weeks after surgery, and take extra care not to raise your blood pressure through exerting yourself for the first few weeks.

Stitches will normally dissolve about a week after the operation, and some may have to be removed after a week or so. Most patients find that they can go back to work after about a week. Residual swelling should ease after four or five weeks. It will be around six weeks before you can exercise again, in particular jogging. Contact the surgery if you notice any signs of infection or have severe pain, bruising, discharge from the wound or a fever.

THE RISKS

- **Implant displacement** Sometimes the implant can move, although it is rare. If this happens, it may require further surgery to reposition it.
- **Haematoma/Seroma** (See Glossary)
- **Scars** The scars from this type of implant procedure should fade and are normally well hidden in the crease of your leg. However, they are permanent and you should be aware that everyone heals (and scars) differently. Talk to your surgeon if you are prone to problem scarring.
- **Infection** This is rare, but if it occurs it is usually treated successfully with antibiotics. If the infection is severe, it may require removal of the implant.
- **Loss of sensation** There is a chance that there will be a difference in leg sensation following an implant. This is mostly temporary, correcting itself as the nerves regenerate, but it can occasionally be permanent.
- **Bleeding** This is controlled during surgery, but it can continue after the operation. If it does, it is usually easily treated.
- **Reaction to the anaesthetic** This complication is relevant to all surgery. Your pre-surgery consultation with your anaesthetist should lessen any likelihood of a reaction to the anaesthetic.

IN SHORT

Calf implants made from solid silicone can be used if a patient desires a bulkier calf contour. Although not common, implanting is growing in popularity. The operation is fairly straightforward but is usually carried out under general anaesthetic. You will be in some pain for a few days after the op. Sensible aftercare is required to achieve optimal results with this operation. There are few contraindications to having calf implants, though smokers are at a greater risk of complications and recovery will take longer. Among the risks associated with the surgery are scarring and loss of sensation. So, as always, proceed with caution. Opt for surgery only when you have fully researched all of the suitable treatments, have been fully briefed and are completely happy to continue. That said, calf implants could be a good option if you are unhappy with the appearance of your calves, as the results can thoroughly enhance them.

FREQUENTLY ASKED QUESTIONS

Q How is the size of implant chosen?

A Before your surgery the surgeon measures the existing dimensions of your calf muscles and then decides on the size of the implant that would be appropriate to your leg dimensions.

Q How long does it take?

A The operation will take around two hours to perform.

Q Will I have to stay in hospital?

A How long you need to be hospital depends upon the size of the implant. Normally, however, the operation is carried out under a light general anaesthetic, and so you will go home the same day.

Q What are the alternatives?

A It may be that that your legs could be greatly improved by exercise and diet. If it is actually your knees that are the problem, you might consider liposuction (page 115), which can be used as a complementary body sculpting procedure to add definition.

BUTTOCK IMPLANTS

We use our buttock muscles, the largest in the body, an awful lot when we sit, but we don't necessarily exercise them. As we age, the skin that covers them becomes thinner, and the muscles underneath become more lax. Consequently many of us are not entirely happy with the buttocks that nature, the ageing process and our sedentary lifestyle have left us with. If no amount of exercise and diet can improve your buttocks to your satisfaction, there are a number of options available to you. If too much volume is your problem, then you could consider liposuction (page 115) to reduce your bottom. If it is sagging that troubles you, perhaps a buttock lift (page 221) is in order. But if you want to augment your assets, then buttock implants (or possibly a buttock augmentation with fat transfer – see page 216) could be the answer.

The buttock implant operation involves placing a silicone implant beneath the gluteal muscle tissue in order to enhance its contour. It is suitable for people who simply desire more volume in their buttocks, or as a balancing measure for people who have underdeveloped muscles or fat in the area.

THE OPERATION

During this operation, you will be lying on your front. The surgeon makes a 5cm (2 inch) incision just between the buttocks and then creates a snug pocket under the main buttock muscle (the gluteus) to the left and right for an implant to be inserted into each pocket. The pockets are made so that the implants fit precisely, and there is very little movement.

In some cases surgeons will use an endoscope to assist with the creation of the pocket to make sure that all bleeding is stopped. The endoscope is a thin tube with a camera attached to the end that the surgeon uses so that they can visualize the implant pocket without having to make as large an incision. Having made a pocket, the surgeon lifts the gluteus maximus buttock muscle and places the implant between the muscle and the fascia (the thick white connective tissue that covers the muscle). Once the implant is in the pocket it has to be adjusted so that it sits comfortably.

DID YOU KNOW?

Buttock implants are very popular in South America, where the fashion is very much for a voluptuous rear. In the UK, they are more often employed to offer volume to people who have been through a dramatic weight loss, rather than purely for enhancement.

The rough exterior texture of the implant ensures that during healing the scar tissue will grow around the implant, rendering it unable to move. Usually drains are inserted before the wound is closed, stitched with dissolvable sutures and taped for protection. The implants are placed high in the buttock where you will not sit on them, so they are less likely to move or irritate.

IMPLANT MATERIALS

Buttock implants come in two types: the first is a solid but malleable silicone, and the second is a softer silicone gel in a solid silicone shell. The solid implant is the same material used to make chin, pectoral and calf implants. The silicone gel implant has a more natural feel than the solid silicone; it will not leak, and even if it ruptures, the gel will be encased by the scar tissue that forms around the implant. The solid silicone implants are designed to last a lifetime, and complications are rare. The gel-filled implants have a limited lifespan, perhaps ten to fifteen years overall.

BUTTOCK AUGMENTATION WITH FAT TRANSFER Another way to augment the size of buttocks, as well as reshaping them, is to inject fat removed from other parts of the body where there may be an excess, such as the thighs. After being processed, the fat is injected using special blunt needles. Only about 30 per cent or less of transplanted fat will survive permanently, so surgeons aim to overcorrect. However, most surplus fat will be quickly absorbed after the swelling goes down, to leave you with a subtle augmentation.

THE RECOVERY PROCESS

As you use your buttocks for so much – for example, sitting and walking – the recovery after having a buttock implant is more inconvenient that any other procedure. When you wake up from the operation you will be lying on your front, and your buttocks will feel sore and painful. There will be some dressings over the wounds and the area will be strapped to prevent the implants from moving. You'll remain lying on your front in bed for at least forty-eight hours after surgery. Hospital staff will help you go to the toilet during this time. There will be drains close to the wound site to relieve any fluid that collects in the area. These may be removed before you leave hospital, or may be kept for several days, should there be a lot of fluid or blood.

The pain should rapidly decrease over the next couple of days. When you get home, rest as much as you can for the first week. You will be wearing a pressure garment for around three weeks. You'll be able to shower properly after the drains are removed, but you must not get your bandages wet. After the first couple of days, you can once again sit during the day, but you must continue to sleep only on your stomach for at least a fortnight after the procedure. Do not undertake any physical activity for two weeks. The stitches, if not dissolvable, will be removed around ten days after surgery.

Most patients find that they are virtually back to normal and back at work after around a fortnight, though sitting will be uncomfortable for around three weeks. Residual swelling should ease after four or five weeks. It will be around six weeks before you can exercise again. Finally, contact the surgery if you experience severe pain, bruising, discharge from the wound or fever.

THE RISKS

- **Capsular contracture** Although implants are inserted via a small incision in the skin, they need a larger pocket to be created by a cut underneath the skin. The body responds to this cut by forming scar tissue around the implant. This tissue forms differently in every person. Very thick scarring can lead to a hard shell forming around the implant, squeezing it into a ball, which can be painful and unsightly. In an attempt to combat this, many modern implants now have a rough outer texture, which it is claimed can restrict the growth of scar tissue.
- **Implant displacement** Sometimes the buttock muscle can move the implant during contraction. Once the pocket is firmly established, however, and scar tissue is growing through the perforations in the implant, it is unlikely the implant will move. Incorrect positioning of the implant can be difficult to correct and will definitely require further surgery.

- **Haematoma/Seroma** (See Glossary)
- **Scars** The scars from this type of implant procedure will be at the top of your buttocks or in the crease. They should fade eventually, although the marks are permanent and everyone heals (and scars) differently. Talk to your surgeon if you are prone to problem scarring.
- **Infection** This is rare, but if it occurs it is usually treated successfully with antibiotics. If the infection is severe, it may require removal of the implant.
- **Loss of sensation** There is a chance that there will be a difference in skin sensation following a buttock implant. This is usually temporary and should repair itself as the nerve tissues grow back in time, but it can be permanent.
- **Asymmetry** No one has symmetrical buttocks and sometimes implants may make any asymmetry more noticeable. If obvious and distressing, it may have to be corrected by changing one of the implants.
- **Bleeding** This is controlled during the operation, but may continue afterwards. If it does, it is usually easily treated.
- **Reaction to the anaesthetic** This complication is relevant to all surgery. Your pre-surgery consultation with your anaesthetist should lessen any likelihood of a reaction to the anaesthetic.

IN SHORT

Buttock implants can be used if a patient desires enhancement in that area. Although not common, the operation is growing in popularity. Unlike calf and pectoral implants, which are always made of solid silicone, buttock implants are made from either solid silicone or a silicone gel. It is highly unlikely that a silicone gel implant will rupture, but if it does, the scar tissue that naturally forms around the implant as part of the healing process will prevent the silicone from spreading. Your surgeon will want to be clear about your motivations before proceeding, and be sure that your expectations of what surgery can achieve are realistic. The operation is usually carried out under general anaesthetic, and you can expect to be in some pain for a time after the op. You won't be able sit down comfortably for around three weeks, and you will have to take extra care to avoid infection of the wounds.

There are few contraindications to having implants, but you can greatly improve the speed and nature of your recovery by establishing a healthy diet and regular exercise regime before surgery. Smokers are at a greater risk of complications and recovery will take longer. Among the risks associated with the surgery are scarring and loss of sensation. So, as always, proceed with caution. Opt for surgery only when you have fully researched all of the suitable treatments, have been fully briefed and are completely happy to continue. That said, buttock implants could be a good option if you are unhappy with the appearance of your bottom.

FREQUENTLY ASKED QUESTIONS

Q What if I decide I don't like my implants in the future?
A Removal of a buttock implant is relatively straightforward, so if you decide that you no longer want the implants at a later date, you can opt to have them removed. An implant will be removed via the same incision through which it was put in, and the recovery will be much quicker.

Q How long does it take?
A You'll be in theatre for up to two hours.

Q Will I have to stay in hospital?
A It is normal for the buttock implant operation to be performed with a general anaesthetic, though sometimes a light anaesthetic with

sedation is preferred. In both cases, you'll most probably be in hospital overnight.

Q What can a buttock implant do?

A A buttock implant will permanently add bulk behind the gluteus maximus muscle of your buttocks, thus creating a shapely contour. The degree of change will depend on the size of the implants, and the size of your implants will depend on your build and expectations.

Q What can't a buttock implant do?

A Buttock implants can only improve the shape and size of your buttocks. They cannot improve your thighs or your figure as whole.

Q How common is the buttock implant operation?

A Contrary to reports, this is still a very new procedure, and quite rare. Just two thousand or so were performed in the United States in 2005. If you do opt for buttock implants, choose your surgeon carefully, to make sure they have enough experience.

Q What are the alternatives?

A Try a sustained exercise routine and diet first, as it may be that your buttocks could be greatly improved this way. In cases of dramatic weight loss, a buttock lift (page 221) or liposuction (page 115), employed as body sculpting procedures to add definition, could possibly be preferable.

BUTTOCK LIFT

If you have been obese and have subsequently achieved dieting
success, you should be congratulated. You made the hard but life-
changing decision to do something about your weight – and you
did it. So now that you're at your target weight, it is possible that all
that reminds you of what used to be is the redundant skin around
your bottom. What can you do about it?

It may be that liposuction (page 113) and a fat transfer (page 108)
could successfully redistribute some fat into your rear to provide
the lift you require. You could even consider silicone buttock
implants (page 214) to plump out what you have been left with
– or you could have a buttock lift. But be warned: this is a complex
procedure and one that requires great skill, so your choice of
surgeon is crucial.

The buttock lift is one of a number of body-contouring procedures
that, although relatively new, can be employed to remove excess
skin and to lift and tighten to improve your appearance. These
procedures are frequently carried out in combination to enhance
the overall effect of surgery. By far the most popular is the tummy
tuck (page 175), but the buttock lift and the thigh lift (page 202) are
increasing in popularity.

> **DID YOU KNOW?**
> Doctors prefer to administer injections in the
> buttocks because they contain few major blood
> vessels, nerves or bones that could be damaged
> by the needle, and the underlying muscle has a
> plentiful supply of small blood vessels to absorb the
> medicine effectively.

CONSIDERING SURGERY

The buttock lift is designed to improve the appearance of your
lower body. When the procedure is combined with a thigh lift, it's
called a lower body lift. If you are considering a lower body lift, the
information found here and in the chapter on thigh lifts (page 202)
will tell you most of what you need to know. With a lower body lift,
you'll be under general anaesthetic for longer than for a buttock lift
on its own, and it'll take longer to get back on your feet.

Like a tummy tuck, a buttock lift is a major procedure and one of the
most painful. You need to be fit and healthy to undergo this
operation, so you will probably have to get in shape just to cope
with it. If you do opt for surgery, you can expect to be left with a
lengthy scar as a permanent reminder of how things used to be.
The buttock lift requires serious aftercare, so before you even
book an appointment with a surgeon, consider carefully the
extended recovery process and emotional rollercoaster you can
expect.

THE OPERATION

At your consultation, the surgeon will have examined your buttocks
to make sure that there is enough loose skin to merit the procedure.
During the operation, he will make a long incision that runs from

hip to hip across the top of your buttocks. This incision is designed to be easily hidden under a bikini. If there is a lot of skin to remove, the surgeon may extend the scar down on to the hips, too. They then remove sections of skin and tissue just under the surface of the skin, and lift and tighten the remaining skin to create a smooth silhouette, before closing the wound with stitches. If it is only the lower part of the bottom that sags, the surgeon may make the incision in the buttock crease and remove redundant tissue this way.

DID YOU KNOW?
If you only have a very small amount of saggy skin, your surgeon might opt for a smaller procedure in which small crescents of skin are removed in the natural crease of your buttock at the bottom.

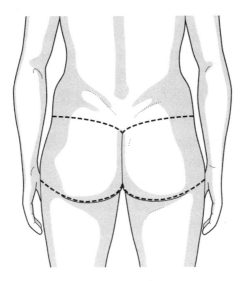

Incision locations for buttock lift

THE RECOVERY PROCESS

This is a major operation, so be prepared for a slow and cumbersome recovery that involves a significant amount of pain and discomfort. You'll wake up from the operation feeling very sore and swollen, and probably numb. You won't be very bruised, but you may feel sick and be unable to go to the toilet unaided for a time. You'll have drains coming from the operation site to take away any excess fluid after surgery; these will probably be removed just before you leave hospital. You'll probably be lightly bandaged or wearing a compression garment in order to prevent clots from forming.

Once you get home, you'll be given painkilling medication and advised to get mobile pretty quickly, though you need to take care not to stretch or strain too much. As much as possible, avoid sitting down or sleeping on your back for a couple of weeks. Stitches will be removed around ten days after surgery, and you'll be advised to wear a pressure garment for about a month after this, to ease the swelling. Most people find that they can go back to work around two weeks after surgery, but it'll be at least four to six weeks before you can return to all normal activities, such as exercising or driving.

It can take up to six months for the swelling to go down and up to a year for scars to mature, so the results of your op can't really be judged for a while. The operation site will probably still be numb: this can take months to return to normal. How you heal will depend on how healthy you were before the op. Finally, do not hesitate to contact your surgeon if you notice any signs of infection or have a high temperature, bleeding, wound separation, a pus-like discharge or heavy pain.

THE RISKS

As you know by now, this is a major op, and you should be aware of the risks involved, which are largely the same as for a thigh lift, so please see page 206.

IN SHORT

The buttock lift operation to reduce excess skin and fat from the buttocks is one of a number of body contouring procedures that can offer reliable and dramatic results. However, this surgery cannot reduce the size of your bottom, nor is it a substitute for a healthy diet. It is a corrective measure most often used following weight loss. Any surgeon will want to be satisfied at your consultation that your weight is stable, you are fit and healthy, you have sufficiently lax skin and your expectations of what surgery will achieve are realistic.

During the operation, the surgeon will make an incision that runs hip to hip across the top of the buttocks, then they will remove excess skin, before lifting and tightening what is left and closing the wound. You can expect large and permanent scars after this operation. The risks associated with this procedure range from infection and swelling to permanent loss of sensation. Although the initial recovery is uncomfortable, you are actively encouraged to get back on your feet fairly speedily.

As always, proceed with caution. Opt for surgery only when you are sure your weight is stable and you have fully researched and tried other suitable treatments, have been fully briefed and are completely happy to continue. A buttock lift could be a good solution to treat problem residual skin left after weight loss; and the results can be dramatic and are usually very successful.

FREQUENTLY ASKED QUESTIONS

Q How long does the operation take?

A You'll be in theatre for at least two hours for a buttock lift, longer if the operation is combined with other procedures.

Q Will I have to stay in hospital?

A You'll almost certainly be in hospital overnight, owing to the length of time you will be in surgery, the risks of clotting and the anaesthetic required. It's most common for you to have a general anaesthetic with a buttock lift, though some surgeons or anaesthetists might suggest an epidural, which would allow you to be conscious (but drowsy) during the operation.

Q What can a buttock lift do?

A A buttock lift can remove excess skin and tissue from your buttocks and make them firmer and less saggy.

Q What can't a buttock lift do?

A This operation cannot give you a more voluptuous rear.

Q How common is the operation?

A Although body contouring is still pretty new, demand for the buttock lift in particular is thought to be increasing. A few thousand were performed in the United States in 2005, but there are presently no comparable records for this procedure in the UK. I have performed this operation ten times.

Q Is there anyone who is not suitable for the operation?

A If you are still losing weight, then wait. Your surgery will have a better chance of success if your weight has been stable for a while and you are within a healthy weight range. If you have any problems with your legs, such as varicose veins, inflamed blood vessels or poor circulation, you should talk these through with your surgeon as they may affect your suitability for surgery.

Q How long do the effects of the buttock lift last?

A The effect should be permanent. However, if you gain weight again after your surgery, you can expect your skin to stretch once again, and the effect of the surgery will be lost. You can expect some drooping of your buttocks with age, though this is natural.

Q What are the alternatives?

A There is a possibility that a similar effect to surgery can be obtained using the thread lift technique (page 275). If the sagging isn't particularly extensive and you have good skin tone in your buttocks, it may be that buttock implants (page 214) or buttock augmentation with fat transfer (page 216) is a better alternative. If localized areas of fat around the buttocks are the problem, it could be that liposuction (page 115) alone might provide the lift you require.

COSMETIC SURGERY:
COSMETIC PROCEDURES

If you can't stand the thought of the scalpel and scarring that come with the operating theatre, then this section is where you can find out all you need to know about everything that isn't surgery. Here we demystify the familiar names you may have come across without being quite sure what they meant, but, more importantly, we also investigate what they actually do. This is the section where you can read about everything from Botox to electrolysis, and from microsclerotherapy to radiofrequency treatment, enabling you to come to your own informed decision about the right procedure for you.

CHEMICAL PEEL

Sometimes the ageing process becomes most noticeable in the gradual dulling of the complexion: the skin begins to look leathery and tired, and deep crevices form alongside finer wrinkles. In this case a facelift probably isn't the cosmetic procedure for you, but a chemical peel might be. Chemical peeling is the controlled burning off and peeling of the outermost layers of facial skin using an acid compound.

ABOUT THE SKIN

The largest organ of the body, the skin is vital for regulating body temperature and maintaining moisture level. It is composed of two separate layers. The tough and resilient outer layer, the epidermis, is constantly shedding dead skin cells. As the epidermis sheds cells, new cells make their way towards the epidermis from the dermis, the underneath layer of our skin. The epidermis is the body's first line of defence against the threat of infection. If it is injured, the skin speeds up the production of new cells to replace the injured ones. As we age, however, the older cells on the surface of our skin stay put longer; this is because the intrinsic processes that cause the cells to shed are slowing down. The result is that the surface of the skin looks old and dull.

HOW A CHEMICAL PEEL WORKS

The chemical peel works by essentially killing off the outer layers of skin, which then peel, revealing new skin underneath. Skin recovers from the injury of the peel by stimulating growth of new cells within the dermis, particularly around hair follicles and sebaceous glands, so that gradually the surface is replaced with new skin. The injury also stimulates production of new collagen in the dermis. The new cells rapidly spread over the injured surface, thus creating new skin, which lacks fine wrinkles and blemishes and has a finer texture.

WHY A CHEMICAL PEEL CAN SCAR

- **Infection** This occurs when bacteria in the wound overwhelms the body's defence systems.

- **Lack of blood supply to the skin** This is most often seen in smokers. When blood does not fully serve a wound, the healing process is crippled, and scarring can result.

- **Picking or pulling skin** If you pull the skin as it peels, you are disrupting the skin's natural healing process, which can lead to scars.

Peels are classified by the depth they penetrate into the skin. The amount of skin removed depends on the chemicals used and how long they are left on the skin. Superficial peels are left on the skin for a short amount of time and consist of fairly gentle acids, whereas deep peels are left on the skin much longer and the acid used is much stronger. Deep peels penetrate so deeply that they cause injury in the upper dermis, which also stimulates the production of collagen, thus improving the underlying structure of the skin. The strength of the peel determines how dramatic the changes are likely to be, but it also determines the level of risk of complications. The stronger the peel, the greater the possibility of scarring.

THE HISTORY OF THE CHEMICAL PEEL

Peeling the skin for regenerative effect has a long history. It was the ancient Egyptians who first used the peeling agents of sour milk, alabaster and honey to rejuvenate the skin. Later, the ancient Greeks developed facial peeling techniques using a combination of limestone, mustards and sulphurs.

However, it was the German physician Dr P. G. Unna who was responsible for the modern era of chemical peeling. In 1882, he reported using carbolic acid, also known as phenol, as a means of peeling the skin. A very strong substance still used today, phenol was used as a treatment for acne scarring in the early twentieth century, and was later employed to treat facial gunpowder wounds in the First World War. After the war it began to be used to peel the skin for cosmetic effect. Since then, the main developments in chemical peeling have concentrated on finding the best combination of peeling agents that offer the greatest cosmetic benefit and allow control of the peel. In the late twentieth century, other agents such as AHA and TCA (see below) have established themselves as gentler alternatives.

GETTING READY FOR THE PEEL

Chemical peels are a delicate treatment. Done well, they can virtually eradicate wrinkles and other signs of ageing, but done badly, they can scar for life. It is therefore extremely important that if you are thinking about having a chemical peel, you seek out only the most experienced and suitably qualified practitioner for your treatment. Before you have a peel, you will probably have some strict guidelines to follow in order to get your skin ready for the treatment. These will vary but, in short, now is not the time to change your moisturizer, book a course of electrolysis, go sunbathing or have any exfoliation treatments, since these can all affect how you react to the peel. Some surgeons will even give you creams to prepare your skin up to two months ahead of your treatment appointment.

> **IN THE KNOW** If you can't stomach the thought of such strong acids on your face, there are a number of peels that use homeopathic ingredients and herbal preparations. These peels are generally offered in beauty spas and are combined with facials. Some of the ingredients in these natural peels include echinacea, mulberry, lactic acid and lavender. If you are nervous about peeling, you might benefit from trying one of these preparations first to see if it achieves the results you are after.

TYPES OF PEEL

There are three basic types of peel: superficial, moderate and deep. Superficial peels are quick to apply and easy to recover from, but the results don't last as long as deeper peels. Moderate peels are better for wrinkles and deeper skin blemishes, but they'll look pretty unsightly while you recover. Deep peels are not for the faint-hearted – they can be painful and very sore – but done well, they will achieve the most dramatic results, completely rejuvenating your complexion, and getting rid of most of your wrinkles in the process.

SUPERFICIAL PEELS

The lightest peels only remove the outermost layers of the epidermis. Often derived from natural fruit acids, and reasonably inexpensive, these peels will effectively treat dry skin, mild acne and age spots, but will only get rid of the most superficial lines and wrinkles. Light peels use either AHAs (alpha-hydroxy acids – also called glycolic, lactic or fruit acids) or BHAs (beta-hydroxy acids – also called salicylic acid). AHAs are the lightest peeling agents you can use. BHA is the preferred peel for the treatment of acne, since this acid penetrates deeper into the oil glands. Another light peel, Jessner's solution, is a combination of salicylic and lactic acid with another substance, called resorcinol. This solution is most often used as a complement to an AHA-based peel. In some cases, a very light-strength TCA (trichloracetic acid) may be used for superficial peeling, though this acid is more generally used in medium-strength treatments.

> **DID YOU KNOW?**
> Light peels can be administered by all medical staff and some specially trained beauty therapists. Make sure that the person administering your peel is an experienced and suitably qualified practitioner.

THE TREATMENT

The practitioner cleans your face with alcohol or acetone to strip it of its natural oils, before painting on the acid solution. The solution stings a bit. It's then left on your face for between two and ten minutes. The skin is then washed clean and neutralized, and you'll be ready to leave the treatment room. Most patients are able to resume normal activities immediately.

THE RECOVERY PROCESS

Some people find that their skin doesn't even peel after such a light treatment, as the skin has already come away immediately after the peel, in which case once the redness has settled you'll be left with glowing and smooth skin. Whether your skin peels or not, after any treatment keep your skin clean and well moisturized, using a soap-free cleanser and unperfumed moisturizer at first.

If your skin does peel, which can begin as quickly as a few hours after a light peel, do not pick at or scratch it or you'll probably scar. If you go for this easiest of peeling options, you can expect any peeling to be finished in a matter of days, and for your skin underneath to look healthy and pink.

The bad news is that the effect of a light peel doesn't last. You should expect to need subsequent peels every four to six weeks if you want to maintain your new, brighter complexion, and you'll have to keep your face permanently out of the sun.

THE RISKS

There is the risk of infection following treatment with all peels, but it is much less likely with a light peel than with deeper solutions. Another risk is only relevant if you suffer from cold sores, as a peel can stimulate the herpes simplex virus. The only other risk is of hyperpigmentation – darker patches of skin triggered by sun damage or sometimes inflammation. A high-factor sunscreen should lessen any likelihood of this.

MEDIUM PEELS

Moderate peels remove both the epidermal layer and some of the upper layers of the dermis. These peels will have a greater effect on wrinkles than a light peel will, they can treat acne scars effectively and they will even out pigmentation problems. Medium peels usually consist of the peeling agent TCA (trichloroacetic acid). Other agents produce a similar result, but a TCA peel is the gold standard. Probably the most common peeling agent, and the one I use most frequently, it comes in a variety of strengths, which allows for accurate peeling. It is very stable and non-toxic to the patient, produces good, consistent results and is extremely safe. Treatments can be repeated if desired. TCA peels are generally administered by surgeons or doctors, though some nurses perform the procedure, too.

THE TREATMENT

The practitioner cleans the skin to prepare it for the peel. The acid itself is applied with soft gauze that has been dipped in the solution or a cotton bud. The practitioner is aiming for a smooth and even application. Your skin will probably swell a little, before it slowly begins to whiten, which is a process called 'frosting' – this is entirely normal. During this stage a fan will be pointed at your face to ease any stinging you might feel. Your eyes may well begin to water and you may wince when the acid is first applied as it can be painful.

The acid is left on for at least the length of time it takes for the entire treatment area to frost. The length of time for frosting can be anything from a few minutes to over half an hour – each layer of application will lead to deeper penetration and the surgeon has to make a judgement when he has reached the desired depth of peel. No aftercare or dressings are applied to the skin after the treatment.

DID YOU KNOW?
It is possible to have a chemical peel on the back of the hands, where it is particularly effective at removing age spots.

THE RECOVERY PROCESS

You'll experience a stinging sensation and feeling of tightness for about an hour after your peel. Over the next few days, the skin on your face, which at first will be greyish-white, will slowly begin to turn brown. After around four days, it will begin to peel off. It'll be annoying and could be itchy, but do not scratch or pick the skin off yourself: you'll almost certainly scar if you do. Where skin has peeled, underneath won't look much better at first: it will be very pink and raw-looking. Be assured that this will soften in time to a healthy glow – it can take up to six weeks for your skin to recover completely.

DID YOU KNOW?
The results of a medium peel last for several years although your skin will continue to age at the normal rate. As this kind of peel does not penetrate very deep into the skin, it can be repeated at a later date, should you require. There is no strict limit on how many medium peels you can have, though your practitioner will best advise you.

Your practitioner will give you a set of instructions that you need to follow to get the best results from your peel. It is important to take it easy for a couple of weeks while your skin recovers. At first, you will be able only to gently splash your face with tepid water and pat it dry with a towel. As your skin heals, use a gentle cleanser and unperfumed moisturizer. You'll probably be given an antibiotic ointment, which you will be instructed to administer several times a day once the skin starts to peel, to help prevent infection. Talk to your doctor about whether or not you can take antihistamine tablets to help relieve the itching, and the same for painkillers if you suffer pain. Make sure that you sleep on your back while your face is peeling. Avoid vigorous exercise for a couple of weeks. Stay out of the sun for at least six weeks, and use a sunblock or high-factor sunscreen when you go out, as your skin will be very sensitive for a couple of months. Contact your practitioner if you spot any signs of infection.

THE RISKS

The risks from a medium peel are essentially the same as those from a light peel, but because the peel penetrates deeper, you're at a higher risk of a complication occurring. These risks include the following:

- **Infection** You are most at risk of an infection developing when the skin is peeling, but if you are vigilant about your personal hygiene during this time, there shouldn't be a problem.
- **Scars** As the peel penetrates deeper, it requires more aftercare and runs a higher risk of scarring.
- **Hyperpigmentation** (See Glossary)
- **Uneven pigmentation** If you have the peel because you have got uneven pigment, it is worth knowing that the condition can recur after a peel.
- **Skin hypersensitivity** This is very rare, but occasionally sensitive skins can become permanently sensitive after a peel. If this occurs it is normally treated with a steroid cream.

IN THE KNOW In assessing your suitability for a peel, any practitioner will want to make sure you are a good emotional candidate for treatment. Peeling is an unsightly business that requires committed aftercare to achieve the best results, so they will want you to be prepared for what lies ahead, so that you are able to cope with how you will look immediately afterwards.

DEEP PEELS

Deep peels penetrate right down to the lower part of the dermis, and can produce dramatic results. Highly specialized, they are usually reserved for cases of extreme acne scarring or particularly problematic skin, and there are just a few practitioners in the UK who actually offer this treatment. I would suggest that you look only for a specialist dermatologist or surgeon to perform this peel. Nevertheless, this is the peel that will banish most of your wrinkles, whether fine, moderate or deep, and get rid of some scars and any uneven pigmentation caused by the sun. But, there is no gain without pain: a deep peel is a once-in-a-lifetime treatment that requires an anaesthetic, and three to four weeks off work before you are back on your feet. Deep peels generally use the peeling agent phenol with croton oil.

THE TREATMENT

Before the peel is applied you will be anaesthetized, so this procedure will take place in hospital. Someone will be constantly monitoring your heart during a deep peel. As with other peels, your skin is cleaned, and then the peeling agent is applied. It immediately frosts on contact with the skin (the process whereby the skin swells a little and begins to whiten). Some practitioners prefer to treat only a quarter or even an eighth of the face at a time, each section taking around fifteen minutes to peel. The reason that this peel solution should be absorbed slowly is that the body will excrete it through the kidneys, and too fast an application would lead to complications. While the peel is taking effect, you may have a couple of layers of waterproof tape or petroleum jelly applied to your face. This will be removed after a couple of days. Be prepared: it is very painful when it is removed.

THE RECOVERY PROCESS

You'll feel quite ill for a few hours after a deep peel, so make sure
you have enlisted the help of someone to accompany you home,
after you have stayed in hospital overnight. The pain is moderate to
severe for some time, with severe discomfort for up to a fortnight
or so, though it is usually controlled with painkillers. Your face will
be swollen at first, and it will be at its worst about forty-eight hours
after the treatment. You will find it difficult to chew, talk or laugh so
stick to a soft-food or liquid diet for the first few days. Over the next
few days, the skin on your face, which at first will be greyish-white,
will slowly begin to turn brown and peel. Any swelling should ease
after a fortnight.

The skin revealed underneath will be very red and may remain so for
up to three months. Sometimes small white cysts and spots (called
milia) can form on the new skin; these should fade with time. While
peeling, the skin will be annoying and could be very itchy, but *do
not scratch or pick at it* – if you cannot resist the temptation, you'll
almost certainly scar.

To get the best results from a deep peel, follow the instructions that
your practitioner gives you. Expect it to be at least two weeks before
you look presentable again. Take it easy during this time while your
skin recovers. You'll probably be given an antibiotic ointment, to
administer several times a day once the skin starts to peel, in order
to help prevent infection.

After a few days, you'll probably be able to splash your face gently
with tepid water and pat it dry with a towel. As your skin heals, use
a gentle cleanser and unperfumed moisturizer. Talk to your doctor
about whether or not you can take antihistamine tablets to help
relieve the itching, and the same for painkillers if you suffer pain.

Make sure that you sleep on your back while your skin is peeling. Avoid vigorous exercise for a couple of weeks. Stay out of the sun for at least six weeks, and use a sunblock or high-factor sunscreen when you go out, as your skin will be very sensitive for a couple of months. Finally, contact your practitioner if you spot any signs of infection.

THE RISKS

- **Permanent hypopigmentation** White patches of skin where the skin has lost its natural pigment are the most common side effect of deep peels. The only thing that can help to prevent this happening is to avoid the sun at all costs and wearing a sunblock or very high-factor sunscreen at all times. If it occurs, it will be permanent, and so you need to consider this risk carefully before opting for treatment.
- **Infection** You are most at risk of an infection developing when the skin is peeling, but if you are vigilant about your personal hygiene during this time, it shouldn't happen.
- **Scars** As this peel penetrates deep into the dermis, it's a painful process that is at the highest risk of scarring. Scarring is more likely if waterproof tape is used.
- **Skin hypersensitivity** This is very rare, but occasionally sensitive skins can become hypersensitive after a peel. If this occurs it is normally treated with a steroid cream.
- **Redness** This is a reaction to the injury of the peel. Some skins are more prone to it than others, and it should fade, but it may take some time to do so.

DID YOU KNOW?
Since the peeling penetrates so deeply, this is a once-in-a-lifetime treatment, so you can expect the results to alter the quality of your skin for many years. However, you will continue to age in the same way as before.

ASSESSING SUITABILITY FOR A CHEMICAL PEEL

All of the following can affect your suitability for a peel:

- If you are sunburnt in any way, a chemical peel will greatly heighten the risk of burning and scarring.
- If you have a rash, wart or infection on your face, it is best to treat this first.
- If you have a history of problem scarring, you may be at greater risk of scarring from a peel.
- If you have red hair and freckles, your skin is probably at too great a risk of burning with a peel.
- If you have darkly pigmented skin, you are more likely to suffer skin bleaching, and so a peel will probably not be suitable.
- If you are being considered for a deep peel, you can expect to have a thorough medical assessment prior to treatment to ensure that you are fit and healthy enough to cope with the peel.
- If you have recurrent cold sores, you'll probably need to take antiviral medication to lessen the likelihood that the peel will stimulate an outbreak.

WHAT CAN A PEEL DO?

- Reduce wrinkles
- Get rid of scars
- Restore a fresh look to aged skin
- Remove skin spots
- Treat acne scars
- Remove freckles
- Get rid of scaly patches or rough skin

WHAT CAN'T A PEEL DO?

- Lift your jowls
- Tighten your skin
- Remove deep scars
- Remove broken capillaries

THE ALTERNATIVES

You might find that it helps to explore cosmetics containing fruit acids and retinol A, which may improve the skin. Otherwise investigate the following: dermal fillers (page 281), autologous cell therapy (page 290), botulinum toxin injections (page 299), radiofrequency treatment (page 268), ablative laser skin resurfacing (page 245), and fractional laser resurfacing (page 263). Of course, if you are looking for a more extensive rejuvenation, there are the surgical options of the blepharoplasty (page 38), brow lift (page 64) and facelift (page 33).

IN SHORT

A chemical peel is the controlled removal of the outermost layers of the skin on your face. Peels comes in varying strengths according to how deep into the skin they penetrate. Light peels will take only the top few layers of the epidermis away, leaving your skin looking brighter, but having only a minimal effect on wrinkles. Moderate peels are the most common: they will remove many wrinkles, age spots and some acne scarring, and will leave your face looking much younger and fresher. Deep peels penetrate to the dermis, so while they are very successful at removing most of your wrinkles, scars and blemishes, they are also the most painful and require the greatest amount of aftercare.

Peeling can take anything from four to ten days. Once the peeling has finished, it is likely that your skin will still look red for a while, but with time it should settle, and it is only then that you will see any results. The deeper the peel, the longer the results last – but also the more potential there is for complications. These include the threat of infection, at its highest as the skin is peeling off, and scarring, which can occur if you try to pull the skin off before it is ready to come away. As always proceed with caution. Opt for a peel only when you have fully researched all of the suitable treatments, have been fully briefed and are completely happy to continue. That said, a chemical peel is a popular solution for the treatment of dull and ageing skin and potentially the results can transform the reflection you see when you look in the mirror.

ABLATIVE LASER SKIN RESURFACING

If the surface of your skin is of a poor quality and littered with wrinkles, or you have problem skin or profound acne, you can opt to have your face resurfaced. Essentially, this means removing the outer layers of the skin to cause the skin underneath to regenerate. If you are investigating facial resurfacing, you have various options. For a long time, dermabrasion (page 273) has been used as a way of manually removing layers, and chemical peeling (page 229) has a similarly long history, but the most recent developments have been in the field of laser treatment.

ABOUT LASERS

Lasers – high-energy beams of light – have been used in surgery since the sixties, but their application in cosmetic surgery is a fairly recent phenomenon. Some of the earliest lasers used in cosmetic surgery are still in use today: these are called ablative lasers. Nowadays, however, ablative lasers are very precise and effective tools, adept at dealing with deep wrinkles and improving skin quality. Essentially ablative laser resurfacing is a controlled burning of the epidermis and the upper part of the dermis, i.e. the outermost layers of skin (see page 231). Direct and intense bursts of light heat the water within the skin to such an extent that it vaporizes both the water and the tissue that surrounds it, exposing the deeper layers of the skin. This accelerates the body's system for repairing itself, so that new skin is prompted to form within the dermis at a more rapid rate, particularly around hair follicles and sebaceous glands. As a result, when the skin is completely healed, it will be free of most of the wrinkles and blemishes that made up part of the outer layer previously.

DID YOU KNOW?
Laser skin resurfacing can be used to treat the following:

- Acne scars

- Birthmarks

- Sun damage

- Skin blemishes

- Fine lines

- Wrinkles

- Scars

TYPES OF LASER

Most skin resurfacing is performed using one of two lasers: either the carbon dioxide laser or the erbium:YAG laser. There is also the Q-switched ruby laser (QSRL), though this is used more often to directly target specific areas of problem skin. Carbon dioxide laser ablation is the oldest and most invasive laser, carrying the greatest risk of complications; however, used by an expert, it has the potential to improve the skin dramatically. The erbium:YAG laser is less invasive than the carbon dioxide laser, because it produces less heat, but it is arguably less effective used on its own. As a consequence, some surgeons choose to use these lasers together: the erbium:YAG laser removes the outer layers of the skin and the carbon dioxide laser promotes collagen shrinkage and subsequent tissue regeneration deeper in the skin.

ASSESSING SUITABILITY

Laser ablation is not suitable for everyone. You may be advised against treatment if any of the following apply to you:

- **Scars** If you have a history of problem or keloid scarring, it might be better to avoid this treatment and opt for a less invasive alternative.
- **Darkly pigmented skin** With this, you are more likely to see changes in skin colour, and so laser resurfacing will probably not be suitable for you.
- **Rash, wart or infection on the face** If you have any of these, it is best to treat it first before inflicting laser ablation on your skin.
- **Sunburn** If you are sunburnt, your skin is already damaged and you will need to recover from this before considering laser skin resurfacing.
- **Diabetes** Diabetics may be at a greater risk of infection than normal. Talk to your surgeon, who will be able to advise you.
- **Resurfaced skin** If you have had any other type of resurfacing, such as a chemical peel or dermabrasion, your skin may simply not be able to cope with another deep facial treatment.
- **Cold sores** If you have recurrent cold sores, while not a complete contraindication for treatment, you'll probably need to take antiviral medication to lessen the likelihood that the treatment will stimulate an outbreak.

WHAT IS THE Q-SWITCHED RUBY LASER? This is a specific ablative laser that is used in the treatment of freckles, sun spots, some tattoos and birthmarks. This laser is targeted directly at problem areas of skin, without causing any damage to the skin around it.

IN THE KNOW In assessing your suitability for a laser ablation, any practitioner will want to make sure that emotionally you are a good candidate for treatment. Because ablation is an unsightly business that requires committed aftercare to achieve the best results, your practitioner will want to make sure that you will be able to cope – not only with how you will look but also with looking after your skin.

BEFORE TREATMENT

Before you have laser resurfacing, it is highly likely that your practitioner will recommend that you follow a pre-treatment skin routine. This may include using light exfoliants, AHA-based creams or retinoic acid preparations to prepare your skin for treatment. You'll probably also be asked to stop taking any aspirin or anti-inflammatory drugs. Some practitioners will conduct a small patch test before treatment so that you are familiar with the process and what healing will look and feel like.

EYES WIDE OPEN Make sure that the practitioner offering you laser ablation is suitably qualified and experienced, and always check that the building where treatment takes place is registered for such purposes by the Healthcare Commission.

THE TREATMENT

You'll probably be given a local anaesthetic, possibly with sedation. Some surgeons, however, prefer to use a light general anaesthetic if the full face is to be treated. Your eyes and hair will be protected. During treatment, your practitioner will clean your skin and treat it with an antiseptic, before applying the laser to your skin. You will probably hear a crackling sound if you are awake. As the energy of the laser passes over the skin, it heats the water within your skin and tissue, causing them to turn to vapour. The laser removes only very fine layers of cells each time it passes over the skin, so deeper and more persistent wrinkles and blemishes may well be passed over with the laser two or three times to ensure a good aesthetic result.

WHERE TO RECUPERATE It will be at least two weeks before you look vaguely normal, so it's probably best to find somewhere to recuperate that is free from prying eyes and reasonably close to your practitioner, in case you do get an infection and prompt action is required.

THE RECOVERY PROCESS

In a word, it's dreadful. Immediately after treatment, you will look as though you have had a severe burn. Remember, the *expected* effects of an ablative laser treatment include oozing, crusting, redness and swelling, so you should prepare for the worst. Your face may be left as an open wound, or closed with a dressing. For the first few hours, your skin will need to be cleaned and moisturized (and sometimes a cold compress applied) every couple of hours. Recovery is slow, painful, laborious and demanding. The best way to heal from laser resurfacing is to prevent the wound from drying out too quickly as that would lead to a feeling of discomfort and tightness. If the wound is kept moist, the skin's natural healing process will be able to work much better.

It is incredibly important that you take every precaution and follow every instruction given to you by your practitioner to aid healing and help prevent an infection from occurring. This means taking it easy at first and being absolutely vigilant about hygiene in order to get the best result and prevent scarring. As the skin heals, the cleaning and moisturizing routine will gradually reduce in frequency, and ointment will be replaced by a normal light moisturizer and sunscreen. Remember, *do not scratch or pick at your face* – it will scar if you do.

You'll probably be seen by your practitioner the day after treatment, then after another two days to check on progress and remove with saline any premature crusting. If you are having trouble with the pain, talk to them about what painkillers, if any, you can take.

Your skin should heal after seven to ten days, depending on the depth and amount of treatment you had. Most people find that they are able to return to work after a fortnight, though you can expect your skin to be red for around six to eight weeks. It is only after around three months, when collagen production has been fully stimulated, the skin has healed and the redness subsided, that you will see any results. After laser skin ablation, it is imperative that you protect your skin from the sun. This means wearing sunscreen every day and avoiding prolonged direct sun exposure for at least three months, preferably for ever.

THE RISKS

- **Blisters and cysts** Since ablation involves burning away the top layers of the skin on your face, blisters or tiny cysts (also called milia) may appear as you heal. These can take a few months to disappear.
- **Infection** You are most at risk of infection when the skin is healing, but if you are vigilant about your personal hygiene during this time, an infection shouldn't develop.
- **Scars** A simple rule of thumb applies: the deeper the laser goes, the more likely you are to scar if you do not look after the skin properly as you heal.
- **Hyperpigmentation** Brown patches of skin that sometimes develop are known as hyperpigmentation. Wearing a sunblock or high-factor sunscreen should prevent them, but if they do occur the patches can be treated with bleaching creams.
- **Hypopigmentation** Sometimes the skin can lose its pigment following treatment. This is more rare than hyperpigmentation, but the risk is increased the deeper the ablation goes. Carbon dioxide laser is more prone to this complication.
- **Skin hypersensitivity** This is very rare, but occasionally sensitive skins can be left very sensitive after ablation.
- **Prolonged redness** This particularly applies to sensitive skins.
- **Reaction to the anaesthetic** This complication is relevant to all anaesthesia. Your pre-surgery consultation with your anaesthetist should lessen any likelihood of a reaction to the anaesthetic.

> **DID YOU KNOW?**
> Your practitioner might recommend botulinum toxin injections (page 299) as a complementary procedure to resurfacing. This is because botulinum toxin impedes the ability of your muscles to move, which actually helps the skin to heal.

IN SHORT

Laser ablation is the controlled removal of the outermost layers of skin on your face. There are two main types of ablative laser: the carbon dioxide laser and the erbium:YAG laser. In assessing your suitability for laser ablation, any practitioner will want to know that you will be able to cope with both the practical side of recovery and also the emotional side, since your face will look worse before it looks any better.

During treatment, the laser is passed over your face, vaporizing skin as it goes. The deeper the laser penetrates, the more potential there is for complications, which include the threat of infection, at its highest while the wound is open, and scarring, which can occur if you try to pull the skin off before it is ready to come away. Your face will probably be left as an open wound that you need to keep moist and uninfected over the next few days. Healing can take up to ten days. Even after a couple of weeks, you will still look very red and there may be blisters, but with time, it should settle. Results should be visible from about three months. As always, proceed with caution. Opt for laser ablation only when you have fully researched all of the suitable treatments, have been fully briefed and are completely happy to continue. That said, although laser ablation might seem an extreme procedure, it can have a dramatic affect on the appearance of wrinkly or tired skin.

FREQUENTLY ASKED QUESTIONS

Q How long do the results last?
A Skin continues to age in the normal way but the results are long-lasting.

Q How common is the procedure?

A The use of ablative lasers is actually decreasing in popularity as less invasive lasers become more and more effective. Of nearly half a million people in the United States who had laser skin resurfacing in 2005, only 12 per cent of that figure used an ablative laser, and this figure is less than the year before. There are no comparable figures available for the UK, but in my practice over the last six years I have noticed a similar reduction of interest.

Q Who can use ablative lasers?

A Ablative lasers should be used only by suitably qualified and experienced practitioners such as doctors, dermatologists or surgeons.

Q What does it feel like?

A The procedure should not be painful if adequate anaesthesia is used. Afterwards, the treated area will feel hot, uncomfortable and sensitive, just like a burn.

Q How long does the procedure take?

A A full-face resurfacing with an ablative laser will take about an hour and a half. Obviously, the less you have done, the shorter the treatment.

Q What are the alternatives?

A If laser skin ablation sounds too invasive for you, you could investigate the new generation of non-ablative lasers that claim to be able to improve the complexion. These lasers do not remove any skin from the epidermis; instead they operate deep inside the skin. Therefore they are much easier to recover from, though they are not as effective at removing wrinkles from the surface of your skin. See page 255 for more details. The latest non-ablative laser uses a fractional approach to skin regeneration – i.e. it only damages a percentage of the underlying skin, lessening recovery time even further. Turn to page 263 for more information. In addition, you can always investigate the following: the thread lift (page 275), chemical peels (page 231), dermal fillers (page 281), autologous cell therapy (page 290), botulinum toxin injections (page 293) and radiofrequency treatment (page 268). Of course, if you are looking for a more extensive rejuvenation, there are the surgical options of the brow lift (page 64) and facelift (page 21).

LIGHT REJUVENATION THERAPY

If you are looking for a skin rejuvenation treatment that is easily controlled, highly effective and commonly available, it may be that lasers could provide an answer. There are different strengths and types of laser, which penetrate at different depths and perform different functions for the skin. There are the strong, short-wavelength ablative lasers (page 245) which literally destroy the outer layers of skin, but because the recovery involved is extensive and is seen by an increasing number of potential patients as too cumbersome, a new generation of gentler light-based treatments for facial rejuvenation has been developed. These treatments use both longer-wavelength lasers and other forms of light as they attempt to get rid of wrinkles, treat skin blemishes, and even remove problem hair.

ABOUT LIGHT REJUVENATION THERAPY

The gentler, longer-wavelength lasers and light used in light rejuvenation therapy differ from ablative lasers in a crucial way: they are non-ablative. This means that they do not remove the outer layers of the skin but instead work at a deeper level within the dermis, stimulating collagen production from the inside out. Whereas ablative lasers simply heat the water in the skin of the epidermis to vaporize it away, non-ablative lasers use cooling agents on the epidermis so that it doesn't get heated and therefore remains intact. This means that recovery is drastically improved since the epidermis of the face doesn't have to be rebuilt. However, precisely because the epidermis is not touched, many of the superficial wrinkles and lines remain on the skin's surface, although these should eventually fade as the skin cells on the surface of the epidermis die off and are shed.

WHAT CAN IT TREAT?

Light-based therapy can be used to treat the following:

- Wrinkles and fine lines
- Uneven pigmentation
- Stretch marks
- Some tattoos
- Active acne
- Warts
- Verrucae
- Spider or thread veins

- Some birthmarks
- Rosacea
- Age or liver spots
- Varicose veins
- Scars
- Sun-damaged skin
- Freckles
- Hair removal

NB Different lights and lasers are suitable for different skin problems.

Some of the most recent developments in this field include the intense pulsed light (IPL), the light heat energy (LHE) and light-emitting diodes (LED) systems. These are even gentler and more flexible forms of light that work at differing wavelengths and colours to cause change in particular types of tissue.

Non-ablative lasers and IPL, LHE and LED systems each make their own set of claims and cite different clinical evidence to prove their capabilities, but they should all be considered carefully before proceeding. None of these systems, at present, offers anything that can compare with the deep facial regeneration that laser ablation produces, though they are effective at treating skin blemishes, some wrinkles and removing hair. That is not to say that in the future they will not be able to. My own view is that currently the results are minimal and better results can be obtained with other procedures that are equally minimally invasive, such as using Retinova cream, light peels and other lasers like the Fraxel laser (page 263).

TYPES OF LIGHT REJUVENATION THERAPY

Non-ablative lasers These lasers have a long wavelength and are lower-energy than ablative lasers. The theory behind this is that the laser heat in the dermis stimulates new collagen production from within the skin.

Intense pulsed light This system uses pulses of blue or red light to damage the dermis, again without affecting the epidermis in any way. The cosmetic benefits of IPL were first noticed in hospital dermatology departments, where it has been used for many years.

Light-emitting diode The LED system involves a light treatment that is a blanket of light over the skin.

Light heat energy LHE is a low-level light and heat system to stimulate collagen.

THE TREATMENT

It varies considerably according to the type of treatment you are having, but essentially you can expect an anaesthetic cream and eye protectors to be applied first; then you may experience a stinging or burning sensation when the light is applied. Afterwards, you may look a bit red and feel sore.

THE RECOVERY PROCESS

Most people find that they walk out of the treatment room and straight back into normal activities. However, follow any instructions your practitioner gives you about how to care for your skin after the procedure to achieve the best result possible. Keep your skin well moisturized after treatment, and avoid the sun for a few weeks, since early exposure can lead to permanent colour change in your skin. If you must go out in the sun, wear a sunblock or a very high-factor sunscreen and a hat.

> **DID YOU KNOW?**
> Light rejuvenation therapy is often used in combination with treatments such as botulinum toxin injections (page 299) or some dermal fillers (page 281) to provide a good overall regeneration effect.

THE RISKS

Even gentle light rejuvenation therapy can permanently scar, or change patches of pigment in the skin, if done badly or if the skin is not looked after well. If the area around your eyes has been treated, you may get some swelling. It is also possible to get burns and even blisters from the treatment, though these should heal and fade with time.

IN SHORT

A lower-energy and gentler alternative to aggressive laser ablation, light rejuvenation therapy is a growing area of treatment for skin blemishes and wrinkles. The range of light rejuvenation treatments is constantly being improved and refined, but it can be broken down into non-ablative lasers (which are essentially lower-energy versions of ablative lasers that do not remove any skin) and other light therapies, such as intense pulsed light and light-emitting diode devices. Since these treatments offer a much gentler form of light treatment, working by stimulating collagen production within the dermis, they are less effective than laser ablation at reducing wrinkles (though they do seem to be effective at treating skin blemishes). Because these treatments do not remove the outer layers of the skin, they are much easier to recover from; in fact, most light therapies can be performed in a lunch hour and patients can usually return to normal activities straight away.

In assessing your suitability for light treatment, any practitioner will want to know that you have realistic expectations of what can be achieved. During treatment, your skin will probably be prepared with an anaesthetic cream, and then the light is passed over the skin on your face. You will probably be red for a while after treatment and blisters could form, but with time, these should settle. As always proceed with caution. Before booking a procedure, consider carefully the claims of what light treatment can achieve, and opt for it only when you have researched all of the suitable treatments, have been fully briefed and are completely happy to continue.

LIGHT-BASED HAIR REMOVAL Non-ablative lasers and intense pulsed light (IPL) can be used very effectively to remove unwanted hair, acting on it in a very similar way to electrolysis. Essentially the laser or light heats the hair follicle, damaging it and thus preventing it from growing again. A treatment can last from twenty minutes to an hour depending on what you are having done, but be prepared for the fact that it can be painful. You may find that the skin is red and sensitive for a time. Remember that lasers can burn, causing the skin to blister, which could lead to permanent scarring. In the same way that electrolysis only works on active hair follicles, light treatment only works on actively growing hair. This means that you will need to repeat your treatments regularly to free the area of hair in the long term. There is still always a chance that some hair might grow, as previously redundant hair follicles become active again or if major hormonal changes occur. If you opt for this procedure, you'll also need to keep the treated areas out of the sun for a few weeks after treatment.

FREQUENTLY ASKED QUESTIONS

Q How long do the results last?

A Because this is a non-invasive treatment aimed at stimulating collagen production in the skin, it will need to be repeated at regular intervals to achieve a longer-lasting effect. A course of treatment is normally spaced a few weeks apart, to allow the skin to rejuvenate itself. You'll have around six treatments to start with, and if you want to maintain the effect you can expect to be heading back for top-up treatments every six months or so.

Q Who is not suitable for light rejuvenation therapy?

A If you are sensitive to light, this treatment may cause a rash to flare up. If you suffer from problem scarring, light treatment could make it worse, and so you might not be suitable. If you are dark-skinned or have a tan already, there are certain light rejuvenation machines that will probably be unsuitable. Finally, if you have an active infection, such as a cold sore, on the area to be treated you should probably treat that first before proceeding.

Q How long does it take?

A Depending on how much of your face is being treated and the

system used, you can expect treatment to last between ten
minutes and half an hour.

❶ Who can administer light rejuvenation therapy?

❷ Most laser treatments are administered by medically qualified
staff, i.e. doctors, dermatologists, surgeons and nurses, though
trained beauticians can use some of the lower-energy machines.
Always confirm that the person who is operating the system
involved in your treatment is suitably qualified to administer
treatment.

❶ What are the alternatives?

❷ You might want to consider one of the latest lasers that use a
fractional process to rejuvenate the skin (page 263). If laser
treatment sounds too invasive, you could investigate chemical
peels (page 231), dermal fillers (page 281), botulinum toxin
injections (page 299), autologous cell therapy (page 290) and
radiofrequency treatment (page 268). Of course, there also are a
huge number of creams and moisturizers on the market that claim
to be able to reduce the appearance of wrinkles.

FRACTIONAL LASER SKIN RESURFACING

Until 2004, there were only two types of laser resurfacing to treat problem skin: ablative and non-ablative systems. Ablative lasers (page 245) work by removing the outer layers of the skin and are a good choice if a very dramatic result is desired, but a prolonged recovery is involved and there is a greater potential for scarring. Non-ablative lasers or light-based therapy (page 255) offer a much gentler alternative, though they are generally less effective at addressing wrinkles. However, a type of laser has recently been launched that claims to be able to produce the results of an ablative resurfacing with none of the recovery problems or inherent risks.

The laser works by specifically targeting the areas that need improvement, leaving surrounding skin untouched, so that only a fraction of the skin's surface is treated at any one time. This fractional skin resurfacing is currently only available using a machine called the Fraxel laser, and at the moment the terms are interchangeable (though new, differently named machines might be available in the future).

Because the treatment has only been available for a couple of years, the long-term effects of this laser are as yet unknown. However, this type of laser looks to have a bright future, as the early results seem to show that it is very effective at reducing wrinkles, tightening skin, smoothing the complexion and getting rid of areas of pigment. I use this laser and have found it to be useful for patients who expect very short downtime and yet good results.

ABOUT FRACTIONAL LASER RESURFACING

The Fraxel laser is different to other lasers, both ablative and non-ablative, as it targets only a fraction of the skin under the outer layers of the epidermis. This laser creates what the manufacturers call microthermal treatment zones in the skin: very small but fairly deep columns into which the laser penetrates. It eradicates the cells that cause your skin to look old and stimulates the production of new, healthy cells that will replace the old imperfections, making you look younger and fresher. A big advantage of this laser is that around these microthermal treatment zones the skin is left untouched, which allows it to heal very quickly.

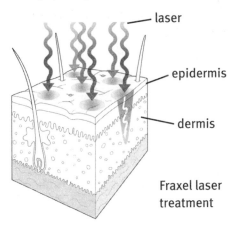

laser

epidermis

dermis

Fraxel laser
treatment

THE TREATMENT

Before the laser treatment, your skin will be cleaned with a scrub to remove any excess skin cells. Then a blue tint is applied, as well as a local anaesthetic ointment. The blue tint will naturally look darker on problem areas, which enables the laser to adjust the level at which it works according to the strength of treatment needed. On one end of the fractional laser machine is a robotic hand piece. This hand piece glides over the skin as it works. You'll feel a prickling sensation on the skin during treatment, but any discomfort is normally well controlled by the anaesthetic ointment. The blue tint can be washed off straight after treatment, which normally takes around twenty minutes.

THE RECOVERY PROCESS

Most people resume normal activities immediately. At first you'll look as though you have been out in the sun too long. Try not to touch your face for a while, and avoid sleeping on your face for a few days. The skin will be red and tight for a while, but it does settle quickly and so you will be able to apply make-up straight away. Men can shave normally after a session. Any swelling will fade completely after a day or so. For the next week, you'll look as though you have a strong tan, then your skin will begin to peel, much as if you had burned your face in the sun. This skin should exfoliate away easily, and using a moisturizer will help during this phase, which will last about two weeks.

You'll start to see the optimum results after around two months, when the production of new collagen in your skin as a result of the laser is really underway. The most important thing to remember is to avoid the sun for at least three months, and always use a sunblock · or high-factor sunscreen in the future, as your skin will be very sensitive at first; if you don't you'll delay the natural healing process.

DID YOU KNOW?
Fractional laser resurfacing can be used anywhere on the body, where it is effective for the treatment of stretch marks, or on areas prone to sun damage, for example the neck, chest or cleavage.

THE RISKS

This is a very safe treatment that has few of the side effects of ablative and non-ablative lasers. However, the following are the risks to be aware of:

- **Blistering** Occasionally blistering can happen if the laser is set too high, but it should heal normally.
- **Discoloration** Sometimes the skin can discolour, but this should settle with time too.
- **Infection** Although infection is always a possibility, the chances of it are virtually eradicated since the outer layer of the skin is not wounded.
- **Scarring** Similarly, scarring can always occur, but if you follow the post-treatment advice, this shouldn't happen either.

IN SHORT

Fractional laser resurfacing is a very new but potentially very exciting face and body resurfacing treatment that can get rid of the wrinkles on your face and neck, eradicate age spots and other blemishes, and even treat acne scars and stretch marks. At the moment the only machine to my knowledge that offers fractional laser resurfacing is the Fraxel laser. As it was only launched in 2004, you may have difficulty finding an experienced and suitably qualified practitioner, though as demand inevitably grows, so will the numbers of clinics offering the procedure.

The laser is attracted to specific problem skin that has been highlighted by the blue dye used as part of the treatment. It eradicates problems and stimulates the healing process around these areas so that the body produces new cells in response. These new cells will not 'remember' the blemish or wrinkle and so the problem will be eradicated.

There are few risks and even fewer reported complications using this laser, but you must take extra care to look after your complexion following a session, since it will be red and very sensitive at first. As always, choose your practitioner carefully, and opt for treatment only when you have fully researched the procedure and any alternatives, have been fully briefed and are completely happy to continue. That said, fractional laser resurfacing could represent the future in laser treatment for the face, and the results attained so far look very promising.

FREQUENTLY ASKED QUESTIONS

Q What can fractional laser treatment do?

A This laser can treat fine lines, wrinkles and crow's feet. It can also treat melasma (areas of pigment caused by the hormone changes triggered by pregnancy) and some blemishes and birthmarks. It can also treat hyperpigmentation (patches of brown skin and darker pigment triggered by inflammation or sun damage), acne scars, general sun damage on neck and hands as well as the face, age spots and even stretch marks.

Q What can't fractional laser treatment do?

A This kind of laser treatment will not get rid of wrinkles completely, nor will it lift your skin, get rid of loose skin or fill crevices.

Q Is there anyone who is not suitable for fractional laser resurfacing?

A You might not be suitable for this treatment if you have a history of problem scarring or if you have very sensitive skin. Any practitioner will probably advise you to postpone the treatment if you have an active cold sore or any other type of infection on your face. Similarly, if you are pregnant you'll probably be advised to wait until after your have given birth and finished breastfeeding.

Q How long do the results last?

A Long-term results are not yet available, but to maintain the effects it may be necessary to have top-up treatments at one- to two-year intervals. Your skin will continue to age in the normal way.

Q How long has it been around?

A Lasers have been used in a medical context since the sixties, but it wasn't until the nineties that researchers began to turn to them as an effective alternative to other facial resurfacing treatments such as chemical peels or dermabrasion. The Fraxel laser itself was launched late in 2004. No statistics exist as to how many people have had treatment, but at the time of writing we have carried out over four hundred fractional laser treatments in my practice.

Q How many sessions will I need?

A Because the fractional laser machine only works on a fraction (usually between 12 and 20 per cent) of your skin at a time, a number of sessions are needed to obtain good results. In general, for a full course, you'll be looking at three to five treatments, between a week and a month apart.

Q Who can administer fractional laser treatment?

A This treatment is usually performed by surgeons, doctors or nurses, and only in a suitable place registered with, and therefore regularly inspected by, the Healthcare Commission.

Q What are the alternatives?

A Apart from looking into ablative lasers (page 245) and non-ablative lasers (page 255), there are a huge number of creams and moisturizers on the market that claim to be able to reduce the appearance of wrinkles. Otherwise investigate chemical peels (page 231), dermal fillers (page 281), autologous cell therapy (page 290) and botulinum toxin injections (page 299). Of course, if you are looking for a more extensive rejuvenation, there are the surgical options of the brow lift (page 64), and facelift (page 23).

RADIOFREQUENCY TREATMENT

Radiofrequencies are electromagnetic waves that travel at the speed of light. They have been used in a medical context for many decades to provide pain relief and stop bleeding, but the application of radiofrequency energy in cosmetic surgery is something very new. Radiofrequencies don't affect the surface of the skin in any way, so radiofrequency treatment is not the choice for fine lines and wrinkles. Rather, it is used to tighten and hoist sagging facial skin. It can tighten skin, lift the brows, thicken facial skin, reduce enlarged pores, address jowling in the lower face and tighten the skin of the neck. When used in combination with other treatments, radiofrequency can also aid hair removal, improve the efficacy of non-ablative lasers, address pigment problems, help to treat acne and even aid the destruction of cellulite.

ABOUT RADIOFREQUENCY TREATMENT

Radiofrequency energy is made up of electromagnetic wave currents. Because the body is a natural conductor of these currents, when radiofrequency energy is applied to the skin from a machine the skin conducts the electromagnetic current and so begins to create an electrical circuit between the machine and the body. When the current meets resistance as it gets to the dermis (underneath layer of skin) on its way round the circuit, heat is produced. Once the electromagnetic energy has transferred to heat energy, it is dissipated, creating a focused heat directly beneath the electrode. This heat can be used to damage tissue in the dermis, which will stimulate the underlying tissue to contract, therefore tightening and plumping the skin as it produces more collagen.

Radiofrequency treatment is a non-ablative procedure, which means that it doesn't affect the outer layers of the skin. In recent years, I have noticed an increase in demand for this emerging technology; with this will come further refinements in technique. I do not perform this procedure myself. My view is that although radiofrequency waves are used in surgery to coagulate blood vessels and stop bleeding, long-term effectiveness in relation to skin rejuvenation is yet to be clinically shown. Nevertheless, I think the treatment is potentially sound, and some practitioners report good results. The most recent development in radiofrequency treatment is to combine it with other procedures such as lasers, intense pulsed light therapy or infrared therapy, which have been found to enhance the results and improve the efficacy of treatment.

IN THE KNOW Radiofrequency treatment is categorized by its means of delivery. Either the current is generated from a single electrode applied to the skin via a handpiece (known as monopolar or unipolar) or there are two electrodes on the handpiece (known as bipolar).

THE TREATMENT

Before treatment, you will need to wash your face and make sure that any make-up is removed. The practitioner will probably apply a local anaesthetic cream to numb your face, which will be left on for a few minutes. Sometimes the practitioner will mark your face as an aid to even treatment. The radiofrequencies are administered via a handpiece that is passed over the skin, heating the deeper levels of the dermis as it goes. As treatment progresses you will probably feel some heat in your skin. Sometimes there is a cooling device or spray that can be applied to ease this.

THE RECOVERY PROCESS

You can expect to leave the treatment room with your face already feeling tighter, but it will be red, a bit like sunburn, and possibly a bit swollen too. The swelling and redness usually disappear quickly, and you should be able to resume normal activities straight away. You may be advised to use certain cooling moisturizers and lotions over the next few days. Follow the practitioner's instructions closely if you want to get the best from your treatment.

THE RISKS

There is a chance that after the radiofrequency treatment you may experience swelling, bruising and possibly some blistering as a result of the heat that has been applied. Apart from these and the constant threat of infection, which should be controlled with vigilant aftercare, the only other risk from the radiofrequency procedure is that 'depressions' may occur in the skin. These are areas of sunken skin, which develop as a result of the overheating, and therefore overtightening, of the dermis. In any case, the risk is only specific to a couple of machines, so talk to your practitioner about this.

IN SHORT

Radiofrequency treatment is a non-invasive, non-surgical and non-chemical treatment that is designed to tighten facial skin. The treatment works by administering an electromagnetic wave into the skin, which will convert into heat as the wave meets resistance in the dermis. This stimulates collagen production and causes the tissues in the dermis to contract, thus tightening the overlying skin.

Recently, radiofrequency has been used to improve the efficacy of other facial rejuvenation treatments. Radiofrequency treatments are quick to perform, and so far there are few reported side effects. You can either have a one-off treatment or book a course. In either case you can expect your complexion to improve slowly after the procedure, as collagen production speeds up. It is claimed that the results of this treatment can last for up to a couple of years.

As always, choose your practitioner carefully, and opt for treatment only when you have fully researched the procedure and any alternatives, have been fully briefed and are completely happy to continue. That said, radiofrequency treatment seems to be an increasingly popular non-surgical option for people who are concerned about sagging skin.

FREQUENTLY ASKED QUESTIONS

Q Is there anyone who is not suitable for radiofrequency treatment?

A Radiofrequency is not suitable for anyone who has a pacemaker or any sort of electrical or metal implant in their body. This is because the pacemaker device could be affected by the radio waves, and any metal present will conduct the heat of the wave, which could be very dangerous. Similarly, if you are pregnant or breastfeeding, most practitioners will advise you to wait until you have finished before having treatment. Finally, if you have any active infection on your face, such as a cold sore, you are probably best advised to treat this first.

Q Who can administer radiofrequency treatment?

A You may find it hard to locate an experienced physician who can offer radiofrequency treatment, as the only people who are recommended to perform this procedure are specialists who have particular expertise in cosmetic procedures and have received detailed training on these machines. Always check the qualifications and experience of any practitioner prior to treatment, as it is in your own best interests to make sure that the person who is performing your treatment is an expert. Also check that the place where treatment is offered is licensed by the Healthcare Commission.

Q How long do the results last?

A In theory, there should be a gradual improvement in the tightness of the skin over the next few months, and the long-term results of treatment are said to last for up to a couple of years.

Q What are the alternatives?

A The surgical option to tighten skin and reduce jowling is the facelift (page 23). A thread lift (page 275) might also provide a lift, but as no skin is removed with that procedure, any tightening may slacken with time. Otherwise, there are a number of facial resurfacing procedures that may stimulate the production of collagen in the skin, plumping it out – investigate chemical peels (page 231) and ablative laser skin resurfacing (page 245).

DERMABRASION

Dermabrasion is sometimes recommended as a procedure that can effectively deal with acne scars, lines around the mouth and other skin problems. However, although it is a form of skin resurfacing recommended by some surgeons, it has gradually been replaced by ablative lasers (page 245). These are easier to control, perform the same function and achieve similar results but with less bleeding and fewer complications. Nevertheless, it is a term that you might hear if you seek advice about your skin, so I've included some very brief information below.

IN THE KNOW It is essential that you have realistic expectations of what dermabrasion can achieve before booking this procedure. In any case, your surgeon or dermatologist will want to know that in emotional terms you are a suitable candidate for treatment, since the recovery involved can be laborious and you will look pretty awful to begin with.

ABOUT DERMABRASION

Dermabrasion involves removing the outer layers of skin on your face. This prompts the underneath layer to produce more collagen, which fills the skin out. It also forces new skin to grow from a depth where blemishes or scars are not present, thus getting rid of such scars and blemishes for ever. However, as dermabrasion sometimes goes very deep into the skin, it can be very painful, and usually has to be done under a general anaesthetic. I used to perform this technique but don't any more because I found it to be somewhat inaccurate and more likely to produce scarring and loss of pigment in the treated area. It is also risky because it leads to the spread of live tissue particles in the air, which can be inhaled.

The surgeon or dermatologist uses an instrument called a dermabrader, which is a drill with a round diamond bit which reaches speeds of 15,000–20,000 revolutions per minute. This allows the operator to shave skin layer by layer until the desired depth is reached. Since this is an invasive treatment using complex medical equipment, only surgeons or doctors should perform this procedure, in an establishment licensed for such purposes by the Healthcare Commission.

THE RECOVERY PROCESS

Once the dermabrasion is finished, a process that can take around an hour, the slow recovery begins. After any bleeding has stopped, you can expect your skin to be raw and red for around ten days. There may be oozing and swelling, too. You will be given strict instructions to follow by your practitioner, and you are advised to follow these by the letter. The instructions may include a careful cleansing routine and the application of petroleum jelly and/or antibiotic cream.

THE RISKS

The risks associated with dermabrasion usually derive from the fact that it can be difficult to judge just how deep to go. The deeper you do go, the more likely you are to cause loss of colour in the skin. In addition, there are always the threats of a reaction to the anaesthetic, bleeding, infection and, of course, further scarring if you do not look after your skin during the healing phase.

THREAD LIFT

The effect of both age and gravity on the complexion is tough. By the time you reach your forties, you will have undoubtedly noticed that the skin on your face seems to be heading south. This is because as you age you lose the fat in your face, your cheekbones become less dense, and the skin thins and collects as jowls near your chin. For those people who would find a facelift too invasive or who feel that the sagging does not yet warrant full surgery, a thread lift might be worth investigating. This minimally invasive alternative lift can hoist the cheeks, tighten the skin around the eyes, reduce nose-to-mouth lines, lift the brow and go some way to controlling the jowls and a sagging neck.

The thread lift works by inserting tiny threads into the subcutaneous fat underneath the skin and gently pulling them back to create a lift. It is a procedure that can be used in any place on the body where a lift is required. The threads leave virtually no scars, are simple to insert and need very little recovery. However, the lift they produce is not as great as with standard facelifting, the threads themselves can move or protrude and the treatment can be quite painful. Thread lifts can be used on their own or in combination with a number of other procedures such as botulinum toxin injections (page 299) or a chemical peel (page 231) to enhance an overall rejuvenating effect.

I do not perform this procedure because I do not believe that it has any advantages over conventional surgical techniques and the results are not good enough. Moreover I have found the results to be very short-lived and the complication and revision rate considerably higher than that of conventional surgery carried out correctly. Still, if the idea of a thread lift interests you, here is what you need to know.

TYPES OF THREAD LIFT

There are two types of thread lift – for one type the threads are barbed and for the other they are smooth. Here is how the types of thread work:

Free-floating cogged or barbed threads These threads have tiny cogs or barbs along the length of the thread. The barbs perform two functions: to provide anchorage points for scar tissue, which will form around the threads, achieving a very secure lift; and to stimulate the production of more collagen along the length of the thread. This thread, commonly known as the Aptos thread, is made of polypropylene, a material used for surgical stitches. With this thread, the surgeon will use a long, hollow needle as a guide, inserting the needle along the length of the planned contour for each thread under the skin. The surgeon makes sure that this guide needle is in the correct position and then removes the guide needle, leaving the thread in place. The tiny barbs anchor into the fat and the surgeon gently lifts the threads, which in turn lift the face. The surgeon then trims the excess thread. Some surgeons argue that barbed threads produce a more dramatic lifting and last longer than smooth threads.

Suspension or smooth threads Smooth threads are generally made of nylon or prolene and can be dissolvable or non-dissolvable. In order to achieve a lift, these threads need to be anchored with a stitch to something stable, such as the scalp. This is a more technically demanding procedure for your surgeon, as they need to have an expert knowledge of anatomy in order to find the neatest place for the threads to be anchored. If dissolvable threads are used, the scar that forms around the thread after insertion will remain and this will ensure that the pull of the lift is maintained. Smooth threads are inserted using a standard needle.

ASSESSING SUITABILITY

Most people who have a moderate amount of sagging are suitable candidates for this procedure, providing they are fit and healthy and have realistic expectations of what surgery can achieve. Any surgeon performing this procedure will also want to make sure that you have enough loose skin, and that it is thick enough to merit the procedure. Unfortunately, you won't be suitable for this treatment if you are on any blood-thinning medication, are pregnant or are very obese or very underweight. Always tell your surgeon if you suffer from problems with wound healing. If a significant amount of lifting is required, it is possible that your surgeon may advise that a thread lift alone will not achieve a good result. In this case, they will probably recommend a surgical facelift.

THE RECOVERY PROCESS

Although you'll be back on your feet within a couple of hours, you should take it easy at first as you can expect your face to feel swollen, tight and bruised. It will be difficult to talk for a couple of days. However, once this subsides, you will be able to notice the lift straight away. In some cases, the skin may appear lumpy at first, but this usually resolves itself during the next couple of weeks. You should start to see the full results of your thread lift after about four weeks, when the collagen begins to build up around the barbs in the threads. Your skin should continue to improve for the next three to six months. Most people have around a week off work for the procedure. If you experience a lot of pain or notice any signs of infection, contact your surgeon immediately.

THE RISKS

- **Asymmetry** The thread can move, which can lead to an asymmetrical result.
- **Puckering of the skin** It is possible that you will perceive a slight puckering of the skin following treatment; this is owing to the fact that, although the skin is lifted, none is actually removed. It is very important that if this occurs you don't attempt to manipulate the threads yourself as you may cause an infection to develop. If it does happen, contact your surgeon who can gently massage the thread and skin back into the correct position.
- **Visible threads** Sometimes the threads can be visible or easily felt under the skin. If distressingly obvious, this may require removal of the thread.
- **Haematoma/Seroma** (See Glossary)
- **Infection** It is rare for an infection to occur, but if one does it is usually treated with antibiotics. In some cases, it may require the removal of the thread(s), which is a more invasive procedure than inserting them.
- **Extrusion of the thread** Occasionally a thread can work its way out of the skin. If this happens, your surgeon will probably just trim the end of the thread. However, you should never attempt to trim the thread or reinsert it yourself.
- **Unsatisfactory result** It is possible that the thread lift will not achieve the lift you are looking for, in which case your only other option is a surgical facelift.
- **Scars** The scars from the thread lift procedure are very small and every surgeon will do their best to make them as inconspicuous as possible. If you do suffer from problem scarring, make sure your surgeon is aware of this before the procedure, as it may affect where he chooses to insert the threads.
- **Reaction to the anaesthetic** This complication is relevant to all anaesthesia. Your pre-surgery consultation with your anaesthetist should lessen any likelihood of a reaction to the anaesthetic.

IN SHORT

A thread lift is a minimally invasive operation that can dramatically improve the appearance of sagging on your face. During surgery, fine threads are placed in the subcutaneous fat underneath the skin, before they are then gently lifted to provide a slight pull in the skin. The operation itself is relatively painless, and a number of advances in technique ensure that now more than ever a good lift can be obtained for every patient. The scars are very small, and should fade virtually completely. Among the risks associated with the surgery are swelling, infection and skin puckering. So, as always, proceed with caution. Opt for surgery only when you have fully researched all of the suitable treatments, have been fully briefed and are completely happy to continue.

FREQUENTLY ASKED QUESTIONS

Q Is a thread lift better than a facelift?

A Some surgeons believe that the thread lift is an inferior technique to the standard facelift, that it is an unnecessarily painful and not particularly effective procedure, and that the facelift is the preferable option to correct facial sagging. My own view is that it is simplistic to assume that threads under the skin will reproduce the results of a conventional facelift, since ageing of the face is a complex process that doesn't affect just the skin; I would compare it to trying to mobilize a paralysed arm with puppet strings. The results speak for themselves.

Q Can I have a facelift in the future?

A Yes. Having a thread lift will not affect your suitability for a surgical facelift at a later date.

Q How many threads will I need?

This varies according to the amount and location of lift required. You can expect around eighteen threads to be inserted if you are after a full facelift, which will break down as two for each eyebrow, two for each side of the jaw, three on either cheek and two for each side of the neck.

Q How long does it take?

A The procedure can take anything from half an hour up to two hours, depending on the amount and position of the threads used. You will normally be able to leave the hospital fairly quickly, though you should arrange for someone to accompany you home, in case you need assistance.

Q Will I have to stay in hospital?

A You will probably be admitted to hospital as a day case only. The treatment is normally carried out with a light general anaesthetic, or a local anaesthetic combined with intravenous sedation to keep you relaxed.

Q How long do the results last?

A It is claimed that the effects of a thread lift can last for three to five years. However, your skin will continue to age, so you can once again expect the sagging and wrinkles that inevitably come with age.

Q What are the alternatives?

A If you are looking for a more extensive rejuvenation, there are the surgical options of the blepharoplasty (page 38), brow lift (page 64) or facelift (page 23). If you can't stand the thought of the scalpel, then investigate the following, which can all have a rejuvenating effect on the complexion: chemical peels (page 231), dermal fillers (page 281), autologous cell therapy (page 290), botulinum toxin injections (page 299), radiofrequency treatment (page 268) and ablative laser skin resurfacing (page 245).

DERMAL FILLERS

Wrinkles are an inevitable consequence of getting older. Fortunately, scientists have developed a whole range of surgeries, products and treatments to help in our fight against ageing. If you can't face the thought of a scalpel and anaesthetic, dermal fillers represent a temporary but highly effective non-surgical solution to problem wrinkles. Nowadays there are so many fillers to choose from that it is possible to create a bespoke treatment plan for every patient. So, if you are considering a filler, this is what you need to know.

As you age, your body produces less collagen. Collagen is a naturally occurring substance that acts as a framework for your skin, bones, muscles and ligaments. As a result, the skin on your face gets thinner and begins to sag and develop crevices, which become wrinkles. There are two types of wrinkles: those created by repeated muscle movement (dynamic wrinkles) and those created solely by the inevitable deterioration of the skin (static wrinkles).

ABOUT DERMAL FILLERS

Dermal fillers are substances that can be injected into the deeper layers of the skin to replace the lost collagen, effectively plumping out lines and getting rid of wrinkles, thereby making skin look more youthful. They can also be used to fill deep acne scarring to create a smoother complexion. There are many types of filler, ranging from natural products derived from the skin of cows or pigs through to synthetic or acid-based products. Most of the dermal fillers available at the moment are short-term solutions that are absorbed after a few months, but science is constantly developing the range. The latest fillers claim permanent, or at least long-lasting, results. Many fillers provide an effective complement to botulinum toxin treatment (page 299), particularly where lines are deep and a dramatic improvement is desired.

DID YOU KNOW?
Dermal fillers can treat the following:
- Acne scars
- Hollow cheeks
- Smoker's lines
- Nose-to-mouth crevices
- Smile lines
- Crow's feet
- Forehead lines

THE HISTORY OF DERMAL FILLERS Surgeons have been injecting substances into the face to fill out the contour and wrinkles since the early days of medicine. In the beginning, patients' own fat was most often used, but this was considered an unpredictable and short-lived solution. As medical techniques became more refined, researchers worked to find a better alternative. By the twentieth century, doctors were experimenting with paraffin, but this was soon abandoned as it often caused unsightly lumpiness and adverse reactions. Silicone was used from around the fifties, but concerns over safety mean that it is rarely used as a dermal filler nowadays. In the seventies, bovine collagen was the market leader. More recently, human collagen has been used, which doesn't require a patch test and will not be rejected by the body. Today, another natural substance in the body, hyaluronic acid, probably represents the safest and most reliable filler available.

TYPES OF FILLER

Bovine and animal collagen Bovine collagen is manufactured from the hide of cows. Once the filler is injected into the face, the body instantly absorbs the saline element, but the collagen stays in the skin, plumping out crevices and filling wrinkles. There are a couple of disadvantages of using bovine collagen, which are the main reasons why it is used less frequently nowadays. Since injecting bovine collagen is essentially injecting a foreign body, you run the risk of anaphylactic shock; however, this is very rare. More of a concern is the fact that around 3 per cent of people will be allergic to bovine collagen. It is for this reason that a patch test some five weeks before treatment is mandatory. However, even if you have a patch test, there is a chance that you might develop an allergic reaction later during treatment. If you do, you can expect to develop hard, red, itchy blotches around the treatment site. In addition to collagen manufactured from cows, there is a product on the market that uses porcine collagen (derived from pigs).

Human collagen When bovine collagen began to present problems, researchers turned to human collagen as an alternative. Human collagen does not require a skin test, since humans shouldn't reject it, although very rarely cases of hypersensitivity have been reported. Human collagen was originally taken from cadavers, but patient and doctor concern about the likelihood of disease transfer led to this falling slightly out of favour. In response, scientists have developed products that manufacture human collagen in a laboratory setting. Collagen was used extensively in the seventies and eighties, though its use is now thought to be less frequent than ever. The main disadvantage with it is that the body absorbs collagen in around six to twelve weeks, so the effect of the filler is short-lived and requires permanent maintenance.

Hyaluronic acid In their search to find the alternative filler that would last longer, wouldn't react and would be effective, scientists turned to hyaluronic acid, a polysaccharide (sugar) found all around the bodies of humans and animals. Some of your body's hyaluronic acid is used as a lubricant for your eyes and shock absorber for your joints, but most is found in the skin, where it is a component of the connective tissues that offer support. Hyaluronic acid is rapidly becoming the filler of choice for practitioners today since it is unlikely that anyone will have an allergic reaction to it and it is more stable, injects very smoothly, doesn't require a skin test before use and lasts longer than collagen. There are many brands of hyaluronic acid-based filler, each with a different molecular size. Some are manufactured from hyaluronic acid found in animals, and some from human hyaluronic acid.

DID YOU KNOW?
Hyaluronic acid is used extensively in medicine, as an injection to provide pain relief from arthritic joints.

Calcium hydroxylapatite A relatively new filler, this is a chemical compound suspended in a gel. It has been used in the past by surgeons as a component for cheek, chin and jaw implants, and it is used by some dentists for reconstructive work. It lasts between one and two years, has no serious side effects and is effective and safe. As this filler is still very new, there is still some reluctance to use it until longer-term effects are known, but the initial results look promising.

Other compound fillers There are a number of other fillers available, and more in development all the time. Most of these fillers are compounds of collagen and other ingredients or hyaluronic acid and other ingredients, added to improve the efficacy and durability of the filler. As the majority of these fillers are still very new, the long-term effectiveness is still largely unknown.

Fat transfer It is still possible for the surgeon to transfer fat taken from a donor site somewhere else on the body into the face, and in some cases this might be the most effective treatment. Fat transfer (page 108) is particularly useful when large volumes are required to alter facial shape, such as for sunken cheeks. Your surgeon will advise.

Silicone Liquid silicone has been available as a wrinkle filler for many years, but its use is controversial and largely unreliable. The best technique for using pure silicone is microinjection, whereby the silicone is injected in tiny droplets. The main problem with injecting silicone is that it is impossible to guarantee its purity, and there may therefore be possible adverse reactions. However, in expert hands, this filler does offer the opportunity of the only entirely permanent filler for wrinkles.

Polylactic acid This is not so much a wrinkle filler as a tissue stimulant. Manufactured from lactic acid, it is currently used as a reconstructive medical therapy for facial wasting, being used to add considerable volume into the face, but it is now also being marketed as a sculpting agent for cosmetic benefit. Polylactic acid is said to be suspended in microspheres, which, once injected, stimulate the skin to form collagen around them, thus restoring volume to the skin. It is difficult to determine if this process will become more widely used, since its application in cosmetic surgery is still very new. Although it requires a number of monthly injections to build tissue in the skin, it has been reported that the effects can last for up to two years.

ASSESSING SUITABILITY

Dermal fillers are very safe and there are few reasons why you shouldn't be able to have the procedure. However, you should not consider having a dermal filler if you have any kind of allergic reaction to a skin test or an infection in the area where the skin is to be injected. Avoid fillers if you are pregnant or breastfeeding, have suffered from any autoimmune disease or have a history of anaphylaxis. Furthermore, if you suffer from cold sores, having a filler can stimulate an outbreak, so be sure to tell your practitioner, who will probably recommend antiviral medication. Finally, bovine collagen should be avoided if you have arthritis.

THE TREATMENT

The practitioner will administer an anaesthetic cream to numb the area, and there is a wait of around fifteen minutes for the cream to take effect. Your skin will then be cleaned and the injections given. Dermal fillers require a number of injections, and so the whole process will be quite uncomfortable. Depending on the type of filler used, the practitioner may or may not massage the area immediately after injection. You may bleed slightly after treatment, and the area can become red and bruised.

THE RECOVERY PROCESS

Most people walk away from the injections and straight back into their normal routine. Once the initial swelling has gone down, which will take a day or so, the effects will become visible. Your wrinkles should have been effectively filled and the skin should now be smooth and taut. You will be given some instructions to follow in the immediate post-injection period, to help you achieve the best result possible and recover quickly. If you had an anaesthetic, you'll need to avoid hot drinks or hot food so that you don't burn your mouth while you can't feel anything. It's probably also a good idea to stay out of the sun and off alcohol for a day or so. You can reduce any swelling by applying a cold compress. If it persists, or you notice any signs of infection or lumpiness, contact your practitioner.

INJECTING DERMAL FILLERS

The injections are administered using one of a number of techniques:

- **Linear threading** The full length of the needle will be inserted into the skin, and the filler administered as the needle is drawn back.

- **Fanning** This technique uses one puncture but alters the angle of the injection as it deposits a number of drops of filler.

- **Serial puncture** A number of separate punctures are made in the skin to distribute the filler evenly.

- **Cross-hatching** The filler is injected as the needle goes into the skin.

THE RISKS

The main risk from fillers is that you might suffer an allergic reaction. This can translate into redness, lumpiness, itching and puffiness. Usually these occur pretty quickly after treatment, but there have been reports of side effects showing up some months after injection. Sometimes these marks are permanent, though this is very rare.

IN SHORT

Dermal fillers are a popular, effective and highly refined procedure that can be used to temporarily get rid of the wrinkles on your face and neck, plump out lips and cheeks or even treat difficult acne scarring. They work by introducing volume into the weakened skin around the problem area. Although they are very reliable, you need to have realistic expectations of what the filler can achieve. The treatment is mildly uncomfortable and can take up to an hour, but results are instant and recovery very quick. The main risk is that of an allergic reaction, which at its worst can cause permanent scarring. Always choose an experienced and suitably qualified practitioner, and opt for treatment only when you have fully researched the procedure and any alternatives available, have been fully briefed and are completely happy to continue. That said, a dermal filler can be a quick and effective treatment that can completely transform the reflection you see when you look in the mirror.

FREQUENTLY ASKED QUESTIONS

Q What is the difference between Botox and dermal fillers?
A Botox (botulinum toxin) is an injection that causes paralysis of the muscles. Dermal fillers are products that restore volume in the skin.

Q What can't dermal fillers treat?
A Fillers won't alter the contours of your face. If this is what you require, perhaps it is worth investigating facial implants or fat transfer as a surgical alternative. Similarly, if you think that a filler is a cheap way of getting something done about your nose, forget it. These are subtle products that can fill wrinkle lines and small crevices, not build a larger nose for one that isn't there.

Q How long does it take?
A You can expect the treatment to last between thirty minutes and an hour, depending on the filler used and the area treated.

Q Who can administer fillers?

A As dermal fillers are non-prescription treatments, they can be administered by doctors, specialists such as cosmetic doctors, ophthalmologists and dentists, nurses and beauty therapists alike. However, the manufacturers of these products recommend that only medical professionals use them. It is in your own best interests to make sure that the person who will be injecting you is a suitably qualified and trained professional.

Q How long do the results last?

A Collagen fillers will last six to twelve weeks. Hyaluronic acid fillers usually last around five months, though some of the newer preparations claim to last up to two years. Each filler is different.

Q What are the alternatives?

A There are a huge number of creams and moisturizers on the market that claim to be able to reduce the appearance of wrinkles. Otherwise, investigate thread lifts (page 275), chemical peels (page 231), botulinum toxin injections (page 299), autologous cell therapy (page 290), radiofrequency treatment (page 268), ablative laser skin resurfacing (page 245) and fractional laser skin resurfacing (page 263).

AUTOLOGOUS CELL THERAPY

As we age, our skin gets gets thinner and becomes wrinkly. This is a consequence of the reduced amount of collagen that the body produces as we get older, an effect that is accelerated by sun exposure and smoking. Recently, however, scientists have begun to apply the theory behind a medical treatment called autologous cell therapy in the fight against ageing. The procedure uses healthy cells from a patient's own body to boost collagen production.

At the moment, two types of autologous cell therapy are available in the UK for cosmetic use. The first and probably most popular is Isolagen. This is not a filler, but a process in which a sample of cells is taken from the patient's skin and cultivated to provide new cells that are injected back into the skin. The other is Recell, which is primarily a regenerative treatment for use by surgeons to promote healing in cases of large-scale skin loss. These are still very new treatments and it is difficult to assess the long-term effectiveness of this therapy, or locate experienced practitioners. Nevertheless, it is potentially a very exciting development in the fight against ageing.

DID YOU KNOW?
The word 'autologous' means 'derived from the patient's own body'. This means that because the cells injected into the face are the patient's own, they won't be rejected or cause an allergic reaction.

ISOLAGEN

There are cells present in your body that have the ability to repair your skin. The number of these cells, known as fibroblasts, diminishes with age, but environmental factors such as sun exposure and smoking can further deplete them. This means that as you get older, your skin gradually loses the ability to repair itself. During Isolagen treatment, a sample of your cells (present in the skin) is harvested and transported to a laboratory, where the sample is used to cultivate keratinocyte cells (the type of cell that is found in the epidermis, or outer layer of the skin). This process will take a couple of months. Once grown, the new cells are injected back into the damaged skin, restoring its ability to repair itself effectively.

IN THE KNOW There is a strict limit to the amount of time allowed between the cells leaving the Isolagen laboratory and treatment being administered. It's therefore in your own best interests to keep all appointments for your Isolagen treatment as you'll not only probably incur a cancellation charge but you could also lose vital cells.

DID YOU KNOW?

Isolagen can be used to treat the following:

- Wrinkles and lines
- Acne scarring
- Burn scars

In the future it is hoped that the following could also be treated with Isolagen:

- Eczema
- Psoriasis
- Stretch marks
- Receding gums

THE CONSULTATION AND TREATMENT

During your consultation, if you decide to proceed, a local anaesthetic will be administered to the area. Then a small sample of your skin will be taken, measuring around 4mm. The sample is usually taken from behind your ear because the skin here is unlikely to have suffered any sun or pollutant damage. This sample, which contains the fibroblast cells to be reproduced, will be packaged and sent to the Isolagen laboratory.

Your sample cells receive their own unique barcode that prevents them from being mixed up with cells from anyone else. The cells are divided and a special environment is created which causes them to reproduce. The process of cultivation largely depends on the quality of the cells in the sample. Healthy young people are likely to have cells that reproduce well, but because the natural number of fibroblasts in the skin diminishes with age, samples from older people may be reproduced at a lesser rate. It is for this reason that an increasing number of young people are having their cells harvested for potential future treatments. It normally takes a couple of months to grow enough cells to provide material for a course of treatment. As the cells reproduce, they are constantly tested to ensure that they are healthy and usable.

After a couple of months, tens of millions of usable cells may well have been generated. When you arrive for your treatment, the injection containing fibroblasts will arrive in a sealed and protected vial from the laboratory. The treatment site will be numbed with a local anaesthetic cream, and the fibroblasts injected into the papillary dermis (the top layer of the dermis, beneath the epidermis).

> **DID YOU KNOW?**
> It is possible to have Isolagen treatment to rejuvenate your hands.

THE RECOVERY PROCESS

After the sample is taken at the consultation, treat the area gently and keep it clean and dry to promote healing. After the treatment itself, most patients find that they can return to normal activities straight away. However, immediately after the injections, your skin may look red, swollen and sore. This can persist for a day or two and is entirely normal. Try to avoid touching the area for the rest of the day, and you will probably be recommended to avoid alcohol or smoking for around twenty-four hours, mainly to help your skin. Don't use heavy moisturizer for a couple of days, and avoid the sun or the sunbed for at least a fortnight. Because Isolagen works by reintroducing into the skin cells that stimulate collagen production, the results are not visible immediately, and vary from person to person. In fact, it will take a few weeks before you notice any difference at all and at least a few months for the full results to be visible. Over the next eighteen months or so, your skin should steadily improve: wrinkles should soften, and the skin itself should become firmer.

THE RISKS

The treatment site may become red or swollen immediately after the injection and very occasionally the injection make cause prolonged tenderness or other minor skin problems. There have also been a couple of cases of hypersensitivity to treatment, but impressively, the manufacturers claim that there have so far been no instances of serious complications.

FREQUENTLY ASKED QUESTIONS

Q How many treatments do I need?

A The standard course of Isolagen treatment is of two injections at two separate appointments around a month to six weeks apart. This may increase if the wrinkles to be filled are particularly deep.

Q How long does it take?

A The treatment session will take thirty to forty-five minutes depending on the amount and location of treatment.

Q Does it work?

A Recent clinical trials into the safety of the Isolagen process involving 1,200 people and around 3,500 injections proved that Isolagen was both safe and effective.

Q Who can administer Isolagen?

A Isolagen is a treatment that can be administered only by suitably qualified doctors, surgeons or dermatologists. In addition to this, all practitioners must receive specific Isolagen training. You can ask to see your practitioner's qualifications at the consultation.

Q How common is the procedure?

A This is still a new procedure, and so, as yet, is uncommon. The total number of patients who have received Isolagen treatment worldwide is estimated at around ten thousand. Because practitioners are required to undergo specific training to deliver this treatment, the number of places where treatment is available is still relatively low.

Q How long has it been around?

A The first recorded attempts to use healthy cells to treat illnesses date back to the early twentieth century, when physicians in

Germany applied the theory in their treatment of thyroid problems. But it wasn't until the early nineties that cell biologists in the United States started to investigate the possibility of applying this theory to anti-ageing treatments. Throughout the nineties, the Isolagen process was extensively researched, developed and trialled, at first to treat skin following trauma such as burns and scalds, before being applied to cosmetic treatments. Isolagen has been available in the UK for use as both a cosmetic treatment and a medical treatment since 2002.

Q How long do the results last?

A There have been reports of the benefits of Isolagen treatment still being visible some seven years after initial treatment, though long-term effectiveness has yet to be measured. The theory is that the injected fibroblast cells should continue to stimulate the collagen in your skin over a long period of time. However, the amount of collagen in your skin will still reduce and so you will still age in the normal fashion.

RECELL

Available in Europe since 2005, Recell is used to treat skin problems such as sun damage, scalds and burns, problem scars (including acne and skin cancer scars) and pigmentation problems. There is even some evidence to suggest that Recell can be used to treat tattoos and that it may promote healing after cosmetic procedures such as ablative laser skin resurfacing (page 245) and chemical peels (page 231), but it is not a cosmetic treatment in itself. During Recell treatment, a 2cm- (^{3}/$_4$ inch-) square section of skin is removed from a donor site in the patient's body; this is then processed and mixed into a spray. The spray is generously applied to the area of problem skin, where it will promote healing and thus have a permanent rejuvenating effect.

THE TREATMENT

Since this is not a normal cosmetic treatment, but a reconstructive treatment that may have some cosmetic benefit, treatment by Recell is restricted to surgeons with qualifications in reconstructive or plastic surgery. A small skin sample is removed with a local anaesthetic from a donor site close to the treatment area (to ensure that the new skin will match in terms of consistency and colour). This sample is then transferred into the Recell kit, which separates the cells and creates a fluid that is sprayed on to the treatment site.

THE RECOVERY PROCESS

You won't feel anything while the sample is taken, since the area will be treated with a local anaesthetic. Once the anaesthetic wears off, however, it may feel sore. The donor site will be covered with a dressing that will be removed about three days later. Keep the wound clean and dry at all times to promote healing. A scab will probably have formed during this time, which should eventually fall off. Your practitioner will advise you on an appropriate skin care routine. After treatment, the effects will be gradual. You should notice the treated area healing well over the next few weeks, though if you are having Recell treatment for skin discoloration, it will take some months for colour to return.

THE RISKS

As with all surgical procedures, there are a few risks you need to be aware of. These include a reaction to the anaesthetic, infection and scars, all of which you should discuss with your practitioner before you proceed with treatment.

THE ALTERNATIVES

A huge number of creams and moisturizers on the market claim to be able to reduce the appearance of wrinkles. You could also investigate the thread lift (page 275), chemical peels (page 231), dermal fillers (page 281), botulinum toxin injections (page 299), ablative laser skin resurfacing (page 245) and fractional laser resurfacing (page 263). Of course, if you are looking for a more extensive rejuvenation, you could consider the surgical options of the blepharoplasty (page 38), brow lift (page 64) and facelift (page 23).

IN SHORT

Autologous cell therapy is a very new but so far impressive therapy that uses a patient's own cells to treat a variety of skin problems and get rid of wrinkles. There are currently two treatments available that use this therapy. Isolagen is a process by which a small sample of the patient's skin is used to cultivate large numbers of fibroblast cells, which are the collagen-producing cells that are naturally present in skin – i.e. the skin's own support system. These fibroblast cells are then injected in high volumes back into the damaged skin, where they begin to repair the skin over a matter of months. Recell is a treatment in which the cells from a larger sample of skin are used to form the basis of a spray that can be applied across bigger areas of problem skin.

Although the early results of these treatments suggest that they are reliable, you need to have realistic expectations about what this kind of therapy can achieve. With Isolagen treatment, the injection is mildly uncomfortable and can take up to an hour, but recovery is very quick and, thus far, no major complications have been reported. Always choose an experienced and suitably qualified practitioner to administer these injections, and only opt for treatment when you have fully researched the procedure and any alternatives, have been fully briefed and are completely happy to continue.

BOTULINUM TOXIN INJECTIONS

Even if you are entirely new to the world of cosmetic treatments, it is still likely that you will have heard of Botox. A readily available, mostly affordable and very reliable treatment for certain wrinkles, it is very much in demand. If you are new to the fight against ageing, Botox could be a good starting point for you, as it is very safe and is ultimately only a temporary measure that won't stick around for too long.

DID YOU KNOW?
The clinical name for wrinkles is 'rhytids' and the condition of wrinkled skin is called 'rhytidosis'.

Many people mistakenly believe that Botox is just a shortened name for botulinum toxin. In fact, it is the trade name for a specific type of botulinum toxin. Some of the other trade names for different formulations and types of botulinum toxin are Neurobloc, Dysport and Vistabel. Botox was the first type of botulinum toxin to be created and it remains the type most often used for cosmetic treatment, hence the large-scale usage of the name Botox. In this chapter, we use the name Botox for ease of reference.

ABOUT WRINKLES

There are two types of wrinkles. Static wrinkles are the lines that reside in the surface of the skin. These form as the quality of your skin deteriorates with age and through exposure to the sun and smoke. Dynamic wrinkles are those associated with the movement of muscles in the face. These are the wrinkles that develop over time from repeated movements – for example, crow's feet (from squinting) or frown lines (from frowning). You move the muscles in your face as a result of a nerve signal from your brain. Over time, the repeated movement of muscle becomes ingrained in the skin and forms the dynamic wrinkle. Botox can rid you of dynamic wrinkles by paralysing the muscles that cause them and therefore relaxing the skin above those muscles.

ABOUT BOTULINUM TOXINS

Botulinum toxins are a purified and diluted version of the toxins produced by the bacteria that causes botulism, which is a serious (and sometimes fatal) paralytic illness in both animals and humans. In botulism the bacteria are ingested and produce toxins in the stomach; these are absorbed into the blood and therefore affect all body muscles, including the heart, causing death by paralysis.

> **DID YOU KNOW?**
> Botulism was named after the Greek word for sausage, *botulus*.

The ingredient that is manufactured to produce Botox is a greatly purified and specific toxin of the botulinum toxin. There are several types of botulinum toxin, each with its own properties, uses and actions. The botulinum toxin used in the cosmetic treatment of wrinkles is generally type A, which is derived from the bacteria *Clostridium botulinum*. This toxin contains a protein that blocks the nerve signals between the nerve endings and the muscle receptors.

When botulinum toxin is injected into the muscles of the face or neck, it causes a temporary block of the nerve signal that comes from the brain to the facial muscle to cause movement, i.e. it paralyses it. The tissues that lie above the muscle also relax, which is what causes the wrinkles present in the skin to stretch out. Botulinum toxin doesn't damage the nerve itself or enter the bloodstream, as the substance attaches itself only to the muscle into which it was injected. Over time, the nerve recovers and once again signals begin to reach the muscles, so the muscles start moving again, the skin lying above it will wrinkle again, and the effect will have gone.

WHAT CAN BE TREATED WITH BOTOX?

Although its use is normally restricted to the top third of the face, all of the following lines can be treated with Botox:

- **Glabella frown lines** The lines caused by frowning, situated between the eyebrows

- **Forehead lines** The horizontal lines that appear upon raising the eyebrows

- **Crow's feet** The squint wrinkles around the eyes

- **Marionette lines** The lines that run from the corners of the mouth to the jaw

- **Smoker's lines** The small vertical lines around the lips

- **Neck bands** The lines that form as bands around the neck

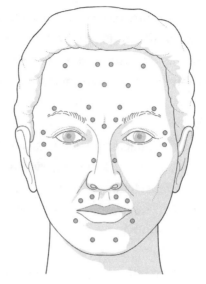

Potential injection sites for botulinum toxin

LICENSING ISSUES

At the moment, in the UK, Botox is still a prescription-only medicine. This means that although it is licensed for a number of medical conditions, it is not licensed for cosmetic use, so, although practitioners are free to use it as a cosmetic treatment, they are liable for any complications that might occur as a result of the injection. Your practitioner should explain the implications of this at your consultation.

A different type of botulinum toxin licensed for cosmetic treatment in the UK is Vistabel. Licensed since March 2006 for the treatment of glabella frown lines only, it is made by the same manufacturer to the same formulation as Botox, but the dose is specifically calculated to treat certain lines.

THE SAFETY OF BOTOX

Botox is a well-established, safe treatment, the effectiveness of which has been proved and which has been used to treat a variety of medical conditions for over twenty years. However, many people remain concerned about the treatment because it is derived from a debilitating and potentially fatal illness. This is understandable, but the reality is that by the time it reaches you, Botox has been through a series of stringent and highly effective purification procedures which make it fit for human consumption. In such a small dose, the effect of the treatment is controlled and localized safely.

THE HISTORY OF BOTOX

In 1897 a physician called Emile van Ermengem successfully identified the bacteria that caused botulism as *Clostridium botulinum*. It was another physician, Alan Scott, working in the early seventies, who first described how botulinum toxin could weaken the muscles around the eyes in monkeys. The first human trials began in 1977. Originally Botox was used to treat conditions such as eye squints, cervical dystonia and cerebral palsy. In the late eighties, the husband-and-wife team of Alasdair and Jean Carruthers first described how it could lessen the appearance of wrinkles. Since this discovery, Botox injections have become one of the most popular cosmetic treatments available today.

ASSESSING SUITABILITY

Although this treatment is very safe, treatment could be inadvisable in the following situations:
- If you are taking any immunosuppressant drugs
- If you have any sort of hypersensitivity
- If you have any sort of bleeding disorder
- If you are allergic to any of the ingredients in the injection
- If you suffer from any muscle disease or motor neuropathic disease
- If you are trying to become pregnant, could be or are pregnant, or are breastfeeding

- If you have an infection or inflammation where the injections should go

You should also tell your doctor if you are taking any antibiotics or medication for heart rhythm problems, as it may affect your suitability for treatment.

THE TREATMENT

Although Botox injections do not normally require an anaesthetic, your doctor may opt to numb the area for you. This can be done with either an anaesthetic cream or an ice pack. The doctor will work out where to place the injections by asking you to move the muscles in your face. Next your skin will be cleaned, the person who is injecting you will put gloves on and the injections will be given. You will feel a small pinprick, but you shouldn't be in too much pain.

MEDICAL APPLICATIONS OF BOTOX

Botox is licensed in the UK for use as a medical treatment for the following conditions:

- Cervical dystonia

- Hemifacial spasm

- Blepharospasm

- Severe primary axillary hyperhidrosis (excessive sweating)

- Strabismus (squint)

- Certain types of focal and limb spasticity

THE RECOVERY PROCESS

There may be some bruising at the injection site at first, and tiny red pinpricks could be visible; these usually subside pretty quickly. Most people are able to get out of the chair and resume normal activities straight away, though you should be careful not to touch or rub the area for at least a day. The only thing you will not be allowed to do following the injection is any strenuous exercise for a day.

You won't look any different at first. Although it is difficult to predict exactly what the injection could do for you, after a few days you should notice that the lines that were treated are slowly reducing. After a week or two, the full effects can be seen. By this point, the treatment site should be largely smooth and free of wrinkles.

THE RISKS

- **Ptosis** The main risk of the injection is what practitioners call eyelid or brow ptosis. This is when the upper eyelid or eyebrow droops. It is normally caused by some of the toxin escaping further than it should. If this happens, there is no remedy and you will have to wait until the effect of the injection wears off for the problem to correct itself.
- **Bruising, headache, nausea** Other side effects that have been reported include bruising, headache, nausea or flu-like symptoms.
- **Double or blurred vision** Very rarely double or blurred vision can occur, and if it does, you should contact your practitioner straight away, as this could be a sign of an allergic reaction.
- **Unrealistic expectations** There is always the risk that the treatment won't match expectations or the under- or overcorrection of the problem could occur. However, a thorough consultation and an experienced practitioner should lessen the likelihood of this.

IN SHORT

Botox is a popular, effective and highly refined procedure that can temporarily get rid of the wrinkles on your face and neck that are caused by muscle movement. Botox is the trade name for a type of botulinum toxin injection derived from the bacteria that cause botulism; it has been through extensive dilution and purification. The injection works by restricting the nerves that create movement in the face, rendering the muscles paralysed. Over time, the skin that covers these muscles relaxes and therefore wrinkles disappear. It is a very quick and relatively pain-free treatment, and patients can expect to be back on their feet within minutes of the injection. The effects are not immediately visible, but will begin to show after a few days.

Among the risks associated with the procedure are headaches, bruising and occasionally eyelid or brow drooping, which, if it happens, should pass eventually as the injection wears off. As always, choose your practitioner carefully, and opt for treatment only when you have fully researched the procedure and any alternatives, have been fully briefed and are completely happy to continue. In general, Botox is a very reliable solution for people concerned about their wrinkles, and the results can transform the reflection you see when you look in the mirror.

FREQUENTLY ASKED QUESTIONS

Q Who can prescribe Botox?
A As a prescription-only medicine, Botox can only be prescribed by a qualified doctor or a dentist. Since May 2006, nurse independent prescribers have also been able to prescribe Botox or Vistabel for a named patient during a consultation.

Q Who can administer Botox?
A Botox injections are widely available but can only be administered by a medically qualified practitioner. Nurses are able to administer the injection, but only acting under a doctor's instruction and after a doctor has seen you to indicate that you are suitable for

treatment. Beauticians or beauty therapists are not allowed to inject botulinum toxin.

Q What is the difference between Botox and dermal fillers?
A Botox is an injection that causes paralysis of the muscles. Dermal fillers are products that restore volume into the skin.

Q What can Botox do?
A Botox can temporarily get rid of crow's feet, forehead lines, neck rings, lip lines, frown lines and chin wrinkles. As lines reduce, you will look more rested and younger.

Q What can't Botox do?
A Botox will not get rid of the lines on your face that form as a consequence of overexposure to the sun, nor will it combat lines that form with age or lift skin that sags. Sometimes dynamic wrinkle lines do not completely disappear. In this case, a dermal filler will also be required to plump out the skin and get rid of the wrinkle.

Q How common is the procedure?
A Since it is unlicensed in the UK, there are currently no numbers on how many people have these injections each year. However, in the United States, more than three million people were treated with Botox in 2005, making it the number one cosmetic treatment in that country. It is believed that Botox injections are the most popular cosmetic treatment in the UK, too.

Q How long do the results last?
A These injections are a temporary solution. For most people, you will see the effects of treatment for three to five months. The amount of time the treatment lasts varies considerably from person to person. Over time, there is evidence to say that the muscle weakens permanently, losing the ability to move as much

and create wrinkles, so you may find that as you have regular injections, you need them less frequently. For standard type A toxin the effect may take up to nine months for the effect to wear off.

Ⓠ Can I become resistant to Botox?

Ⓐ It is possible to become resistant to the injection over time. It is estimated that between 1 and 2 per cent of people will develop antibodies that block the effects of the treatment, rendering it useless. In these cases, a different strain of botulinum toxin could be an alternative.

Ⓠ How long does it take?

Ⓐ The treatment can take twenty to thirty minutes depending on the amount and location of the injections.

Ⓠ What are the alternatives?

Ⓐ There are a huge number of creams and moisturizers on the market that claim to be able to reduce the appearance of wrinkles. Otherwise, investigate the thread lift (page 275), chemical peels (page 231), dermal fillers (page 281), autologous cell therapy (page 290), radiofrequency treatment (page 268), ablative laser skin resurfacing (page 245) and fractional laser skin resurfacing (page 263). Of course, if you are looking for a more extensive rejuvenation, there are the surgical options of the blepharoplasty (page 38), brow lift (page 64) and facelift (page 23).

SCLEROTHERAPY AND MICRO-THERMOCOAGULATION

Thread veins can be inherited or brought on by trauma, pregnancy or weight gain. Most often found on the face and legs, they are easily noticeable as tiny red, blue or purple veins that can be seen through the skin. More than 50 per cent of women are said to suffer from them. For many, although unsightly, they present no medical problem, apart from perhaps aching occasionally, and so they are left untouched. However, there are a number of treatments that claim to be able to improve the appearance of thread veins.

One of the most popular procedures, and still regarded by many practitioners as the treatment of choice, is called *sclerotherapy* or *microsclerotherapy*. Strictly speaking, sclerotherapy is the term used for treatment of larger veins, and microsclerotherapy is the term generally used for tiny thread veins, but today the terms are somewhat interchangeable. The other interesting treatment for thread veins is called *micro-thermocoagulation*, which is a new treatment that utilizes microwaves to collapse the vein.

SCLEROTHERAPY

Sclerotherapy involves injecting the veins with a sclerosant solution designed to damage the lining of these blood vessels, so that they collapse and disappear. Reserved for leg thread veins, it is not used for facial thread veins because of the risk of scarring. My own view of sclerotherapy is that it is an excellent treatment for getting rid of thread veins on the legs, although the results are entirely dependent on the practitioner.

KNOW YOUR VEINS

- **Veins** These are the channels by which deoxygenated blood is carried back to the heart.

- **Thread veins and spider veins** These are tiny veins that begin to show through the surface of the skin as a result of increased pressure in the vein. They are usually just a few millimetres across.

- **Varicose veins** Rope-like bulging veins on the legs, which can be very painful, these are a separate medical problem. A specialist vascular surgeon usually treats varicose veins.

THE TREATMENT

Once the area for treatment has been cleaned with antiseptic, the practitioner will stretch the skin of the area to be injected and then inject the solution into the veins one at a time, depending upon how long they are. You shouldn't feel any pain, but you may feel a slight stinging or burning sensation. After the injection, a cotton wool ball will be taped over the veins to aid healing. You will be instructed to wear a compression garment on your legs to ease any swelling and to aid healing.

THE RECOVERY PROCESS

Most patients find that they can get up and resume normal activities straight away, though it is probably a good idea to take it easy and elevate your legs as much as possible at first – your practitioner will advise you. However, you can expect some discomfort after the procedure. Among the normal consequences of treatment are leg cramps, bruising, swelling and tenderness. In addition, you will have to be emotionally prepared for the recovery process as your legs will look worse before they look any better.

The swabs and compression garment placed on your legs after treatment will remain in place for at least forty-eight hours; many practitioners will suggest longer. After around three days, if the garment has come off, you can expect the treatment area to look bruised, often like insect bites, and swollen. You can also expect your legs to cramp or be itchy. Talk to your practitioner about what, if any, painkillers you can take to ease this, and remember to be vigilant for signs of infection. Contact the treatment clinic if you think the area may be infected.

Once the initial recovery period is over, you should aim to get mobile fairly quickly to avoid the possibility of clots forming in your legs, but stick to walking and gentle exercise until your practitioner says that it is safe to do more. In the future, you should keep the treated area out of the sun. The veins will look quite bad for a few weeks, but they should gradually fade until they are almost completely clear after a month. It will take several months before the final result becomes apparent. In some cases a patch of brown discoloration can persist and can take up to a year to fade completely.

IN THE KNOW Plan your sclerotherapy well in advance of any travelling you are likely to do, as you are advised not to go on a long-haul flight for at least two weeks before or after your treatment.

THE RISKS

You should be aware of the following risks:

- **Ulcers/scars** Sometimes small ulcers can develop around the treatment site. These ulcers can leave small scars when they have healed.
- **Blood clots** Although extremely rare, this complication has been reported after treatment.
- **Swelling** Sometimes the swelling that is normal after the procedure can persist or get worse. Swelling can also occur if some of the sclerosant solution escapes from the vein.
- **Allergic response** There is always a possibility of an allergic response to the sclerosant solution, although this is very unlikely.
- **Hyperpigmentation** (See Glossary)
- **Tissue necrosis** (See Glossary)
- **Spider vein matting** There are occasions when reddish blood vessels develop around the treatment site. If this happens, further injections may be required.

DID YOU KNOW?

Sclerotherapy is not advised if you are pregnant or breastfeeding, diabetic, or taking steroid medication.

IN SHORT

Sclerotherapy is a popular and highly refined procedure that can reduce the appearance of thread veins on your legs. The treatment works by injecting a sclerosant solution into the vein, causing damage that eventually makes the vein disappear. After treatment the area may be a bit red and swollen, but this will quickly pass.

FREQUENTLY ASKED QUESTIONS

Q What is in the sclerosant solution?

A There are two types of products that are injected into spider veins: detergents and hypertonic solutions. Detergents work by destroying the proteins in the cell membrane, causing it to die. Hypertonics work by dehydrating the cells, causing the vein to collapse.

Q Who can administer treatment?

A The manufacturers of sclerosant solutions recommend that only medically qualified practitioners perform sclerotherapy, and therefore beauty therapists should not. However, it is still the case that sometimes specially trained therapists offer the procedure. It is always in your own best interest to seek out the most suitably qualified and competent practitioner for your treatment. There are many general practitioners, nurses and dermatologists who can perform the treatment and it may well be that they are more experienced.

Q How many treatments will I need?

A Thread veins have a tendency to come back, so you can expect to need more than one treatment if permanent removal is required. The average course of sclerotherapy is four to six sessions, usually spaced about a month apart, allowing time for the skin to settle. The thread veins should progressively get better during the course. Once the course is finished, you might still have to return again, as thread veins can persist.

Q How long does it take?

A This depends upon the number of thread veins you are having treated, but in general a sclerotherapy session lasts for up to forty separate injections, which would take about forty-five minutes.

Q How long has the procedure been around?

A Sclerotherapy treatment was pioneered in the twenties as a treatment for varicose veins, before being refined to treat thread veins.

MICRO-THERMOCOAGULATION

Micro-thermocoagulation treatment works by applying microwaves directly into the thread vein via a very fine insulated needle, which in turn heats the capillary to such an extent that it causes the vein to collapse, thus making the thread vein disappear. The needle is so small it is unable to damage any of the surrounding tissue. It is claimed that micro-thermocoagulation treatment can reduce facial and leg thread veins on any skin type, and also treat some psoriasis and rosacea. At the moment, one trade name that is associated with this procedure is Veinwave.

THE TREATMENT

The treatment machine is an instrument that has what looks like a pen on one end: this is where the needle is attached. This needle, which should be sterile and used only once for your treatment, is inserted into the vein and the machine is switched on. The needle heats up very quickly as the wave is administered, and the machine is then switched off. You should only feel a tiny amount of pressure during treatment and in theory the thread vein should start to disappear instantaneously, although it will be a couple of days before the full results of the treatment will show.

THE RECOVERY PROCESS

You can expect to see a few red marks and perhaps some tiny scabs after treatment, but these should heal and fall off within a couple of days. However, it is possible that new thread veins could develop in the area that was treated, or even in an entirely new area in the future. So although this treatment can be very effective, you may well find that you need to return for more treatments at a later date.

IN THE KNOW If you have a pacemaker or are epileptic, you won't be able to have this treatment. If you are pregnant or breastfeeding, you will probably be advised to wait until after you have finished nursing before considering treatment.

DID YOU KNOW?
It might be worth paying a visit to your GP to rule out any underlying condition before you book this treatment, as thread veins can be a sign of a problem with your circulation.

THE RISKS

There is a very small risk of scarring, and there is always the threat of infection to consider, but as yet there do not seem to have been any reports of other complications from this procedure. Taking extra care to make sure that the treatment site remains clean after the procedure should reduce any chance of an infection developing. There is no risk of burning from the needle as it is heat-insulated.

IN SHORT

With micro-thermocoagulation, a microwave current is passed into the vein to collapse it, thus making the vein disappear. During the treatment, a fine insulated needle is passed into the vein and the current administered. Some scabs may form after treatment, but these should quickly fall away. As always, opt for the treatment most suitable to you only when you have fully researched the procedure and any alternatives, have been fully briefed and are completely happy to continue.

FREQUENTLY ASKED QUESTIONS

Q Who can administer treatment?

A Micro-thermocoagulation should only be carried out by suitably qualified and experienced doctors, surgeons and some specially trained nurses.

Q How many treatments will I need?

A With micro-thermocoagulation, how many sessions you require is usually dependent on the size and location of the treatment area. Many people find that one session does the trick, but your practitioner may recommend a course to achieve a better result.

Q How long does it take?

A A session of micro-thermocoagulation usually involves over two hundred pulses and lasts about fifteen minutes. Around 40cm (16 inches) of thread veins can be treated during that time.

Q How long has the procedure been around?

A Micro-thermocoagulation in the form of the Veinwave treatment has been used in the UK since 2001.

Q What are the alternatives?

A My own view is that treatment of thread veins, especially facial ones, is perhaps best done by specific lasers, which are both safe and very effective.

ELECTROLYSIS

If you suffer from excess hair and you are looking for a more permanent way of getting rid of it, your options include laser treatment, intense pulsed light treatment and electrolysis. Electrolysis is a form of permanent hair reduction that uses heat and electricity to destroy the skin's capacity to grow hair in the treated follicles. However, permanent hair removal can be a slow and cumbersome business, as each hair follicle is treated individually. Be prepared for repeat treatments and a certain amount of pain before getting to be permanently free of hair in a given area.

ABOUT YOUR HAIR

Each hair on your body usually grows from a single follicle (although occasionally two or three can grow from the same spot). The follicle has its own blood and nerve supply, and it is the blood capillaries around the follicle that provide the base of the follicle, the papilla, with all it needs to grow. Electrolysis damages the connection between the supply of nourishments from the blood to the hair follicle, thus disabling the follicle from growing new hair.

TYPES OF ELECTROLYSIS

Galvanic electrolysis The original method, this used a direct current of electricity. The electricity, when combined with the skin's natural water and salt in the hair follicle, produces a chemical compound that damages the cells that cause hair growth.

Thermolysis Also called diathermy or short-wave electrolysis, this uses an alternating current of electricity. The current creates heat in the follicle, which damages it, rendering it unable to grow.

Blend electrolysis This is a mixture of the two procedures. The heat and chemical compound are used in combination to destroy the hair follicle.

WHAT AREAS CAN BE TREATED?

The only places that can't be treated with electrolysis are the hair inside the nose and ears. Some of the most popular places for treatment are:

• Bikini line	• Chest	• Fingers
• Legs	• Nipples	• Lips
• Toes	• Abdomen	• Chin
• Backs of thighs	• Back	• Nose
• Hairline	• Underarms	• Sides of face
• Rims of ears	• Arms	• Neck
• Eyebrows	• Hands	

THE TREATMENT

During treatment, the practitioner inserts a tiny probe directly into the hair follicle. You shouldn't feel this, as the needle is so small that it shouldn't damage the skin. Once inserted, an electric current is sent into the follicle to destroy the hair. There are usually a couple of seconds of pain while the current works, like a sting. Any loose hairs left after the current has worked are removed with tweezers.

Although electrolysis is a method of permanent hair reduction, this treatment only works on follicles that are growing hair at that time of the procedure. Therefore, as other follicles become active, repeat treatments will be needed to ensure complete hair removal. Treatments will probably take place once a week at first. Individual sessions can last for anything from a few minutes right up to two hours, depending on what is being treated and how much you can tolerate in a session. Once you begin the course, you will find that the need for treatment will become more infrequent as the hair growth slows. Hair removal on smaller areas, such as the chin, can take as little as a couple of hours, while more demanding areas, such as the bikini line, can take up to sixteen hours.

THE RISKS

Performed by an expert, electrolysis treatment has very few risks. You can expect the area to be red and swollen for a short while after a session, but this should fade quickly. Sometimes whiteheads and scabs can develop, and if this happens, try to avoid picking them or you could scar. There is always the possibility of infection. Also, you can be left with permanent scars from this procedure if it is done badly.

IN SHORT

Electrolysis is a popular and highly refined procedure that can permanently reduce problem hair on both your face and body. The treatment works by passing an electric current into the hair follicle and causing damage that permanently stops the follicle from growing hair. There are three types of electrolysis and your practitioner will advise as to the best option in your case. You can expect to undergo regular sessions lasting anything from a few minutes to a couple of hours at a time. After treatment the area will be red and swollen, but this will quickly pass. As always, opt for treatment only when you have fully researched the procedure and any alternatives, have been fully briefed and are completely happy to continue.

> **DID YOU KNOW?**
> Hair grows at a rate of around 12mm (½ inch) a month and is faster in summer than in winter. This is because the level of androgen hormone peaks in summer, stimulating hair growth.

FREQUENTLY ASKED QUESTIONS

Q Who can administer electrolysis?

A While members of the medical profession and appropriately trained beauty therapists can perform electrolysis, it is in your own best interest to seek the most suitably trained and experienced practitioners.

Q What is the recovery process like?

A Most people find that they are able to continue with normal activities immediately. You should take care not to touch the treated area too much at first and wear sunblock to protect your skin.

Q How long has it been around?

A In 1875, an American physician called Charles E. Michel first reported permanently removing hair using an electric current. Originally it was used as treatment to destroy ingrowing eyelashes.

Q What are the alternatives?

A It's back to sugaring, shaving, waxing, cream depilatories or plucking for temporary removal of hair. However, if permanent hair removal remains your goal, you could investigate light-based hair removal (page 255).

COSMETIC SURGERY:
USEFUL REFERENCES

Once you've learned all about the surgery and procedures, you need to know what to consider next. With this in mind, I have put together a section consisting of everything else you need to understand as you investigate cosmetic surgery for yourself. Starting with a guide to all the associations and websites you should check out as part of your research, I then offer my own guide to finding the right cosmetic surgeon for you. There is also a useful guide to demystifying some of the medical qualifications you should be aware of, and information about cosmetic surgery abroad. At the end of this section, I have included an accessible glossary of commonly used terms that you can refer to whenever all that technical and medical jargon gets too much.

COSMETIC SURGERY CONTACTS, USEFUL WEBSITES AND FURTHER INFORMATION

THE DEPARTMENT OF HEALTH
INFORMATION AND GUIDANCE ON
COSMETIC SURGERY
www.dh.gov.uk/cosmeticsurgery
The Department of Health
Richmond House, 79 Whitehall
London SW1A 2NS
020 7210 4850

HEALTHCARE COMMISSION
http://www.healthcarecommission.org.uk/
Head Office – London
Finsbury Tower, 103–105 Bunhill Row
London EC1Y 8TG
020 7448 9200

Bristol
Dominions House, Lime Kiln Close
Stoke Gifford, Bristol BS34 8SR
020 7448 8158

Leeds
Kernel House, Killingbeck Drive
Killingbeck, Leeds LS14 6UF
020 7448 8179

Manchester
5th Floor, Peter House, Oxford Street
Manchester M1 5AX
020 7448 9100

Nottingham
Maid Marian House, 56 Hounds Gate
Nottingham NG1 6BG
020 7448 8188

Solihull
1st Floor, 1 Friarsgate, 1011 Stratford
Road, Solihull B90 4AG
020 7448 9200

THE GENERAL MEDICAL COUNCIL
http://www.gmc-uk.org/
0845 357 3456

London
Regent's Place, 350 Euston Road
London NW1 3JN

Manchester
St James's Buildings, 79 Oxford Street
Manchester M1 6FQ

Edinburgh
Napier House, 35 Thistle Street
Edinburgh EH2 1DY

Cardiff
Regus House, Falcon Drive
Cardiff Bay CF10 4RU

Belfast
20 Adelaide Street, Belfast BT2 8GB

BRITISH ASSOCIATION OF AESTHETIC PLASTIC SURGEONS
www.baaps.org.uk/
at the Royal College of Surgeons
of England
35–43 Lincoln's Inn Fields
London WC2A 3PE
020 7405 2234

THE BRITISH ASSOCIATION OF COSMETIC SURGEONS
http://www.b-a-c-s.co.uk/bacs.htm
Highgate Private Hospital
17–19 View Road, Highgate
London N6 4DJ

THE BRITISH ASSOCIATION OF COSMETIC DOCTORS
http://www.cosmeticdoctors.co.uk/
30b Wimpole Street
London W1U 2RW
0800 328 3613

THE BRITISH ASSOCIATION OF PLASTIC, RECONSTRUCTIVE AND AESTHETIC SURGEONS
http://www.bapras.org.uk/
at the Royal College of Surgeons
35–43 Lincoln's Inn Fields
London WC2A 3PE
020 7831 5161

THE BRITISH ASSOCIATION OF DERMATOLOGISTS

www.bad.org.uk
4 Fitzroy Square, London W1T 5HQ
020 7383 0266

THE BRITISH MEDICAL ASSOCIATION
http://www.bma.org.uk/
BMA House, Tavistock Square
London WC1H 9JP
020 7387 4499

THE ROYAL COLLEGE OF SURGEONS OF ENGLAND
http://www.rcseng.ac.uk/
35–43 Lincoln's Inn Fields
London WC2A 3PE
020 7405 3474

THE ROYAL COLLEGE OF SURGEONS OF ENGLAND PATIENT LIAISON GROUP
http://www.rcseng.ac.uk/patient_ information/plg
35–43 Lincoln's Inn Fields
London WC2A 3PE
020 7405 3474

ROYAL COLLEGE OF ANAESTHETISTS
http://www.rcoa.ac.uk/
Churchill House, 35 Red Lion Square
London WC1R 4SG
020 7092 1500

ROYAL COLLEGE OF PHYSICIANS
http://www.rcplondon.ac.uk/
11 St Andrews Place, Regent's Park
London NW1 4LE
020 7935 1174

ROYAL COLLEGE OF NURSING
http://www.rcn.org.uk/
20 Cavendish Square
London W1G 0RN
020 7409 3333

THE ROYAL COLLEGE OF OPHTHALMOLOGISTS
http://www.rcophth.ac.uk/
17 Cornwall Terrace
London NW1 4QW
020 7935 0702

NURSING AND MIDWIFERY COUNCIL
http://www.nmc-uk.org/
Nursing and Midwifery Council
23 Portland Place, London W1B 1PZ
020 7637 7181

THE ASSOCIATION OF ANAESTHETISTS OF GREAT BRITAIN AND IRELAND
http://www.aagbi.org/
21 Portland Place, London W1B 1PY
0207 631 1650

THE INSTITUTE OF COSMETIC AND RECONSTRUCTIVE SURGERY
http://www.icr-surgery.com/
1 Parkside, Ravenscourt Park
London W6 0UU
020 8735 6063

MEDICINES AND HEALTHCARE PRODUCTS REGULATORY AGENCY (MHRA)
http://www.mhra.gov.uk/
Information Centre, 10–12 Market Towers, 1 Nine Elms Lane
London SW8 5NQ
020 7084 2000
020 7210 3000

NHS DIRECT ONLINE
http://www.nhsdirect.nhs.uk/
0845 4647

THE PATIENTS ASSOCIATION
http://www.patients-association.org.uk/
PO Box 935, Harrow

Middlesex HA1 3YJ
0845 608 4455

PATIENT ADVISORY SERVICE
http://www.patientadvisory.co.uk/location.htm
136 Harley Street, London W1G
0800 033 6024

MEDICAL ADVISORY SERVICE
http://www.medicaladvisoryservice.org.uk/
020 8995 8503

PATIENT ADVICE AND LIAISON SERVICE
http://www.pals.nhs.uk/
Suite 24, Beechfield House
Lyme Green Business Park
Winterton Way, Macclesfield
Cheshire SK11 0LP
01625 509155

THE INDEPENDENT SECTOR COMPLAINTS ADJUDICATION SERVICE
Centre Point, 103 New Oxford Street
London WC1A IDU
020 7379 8598

ACTION FOR VICTIMS OF MEDICAL ACCIDENTS
http://www.avma.org.uk/
44 High Street, Croydon
Surrey CR0 1YB
0845 123 2352

THE INDEPENDENT HEALTHCARE FORUM
http://www.independenthealthcare.org.uk/
Centre Point, 103 New Oxford Street
London WC1A IDU
020 7379 8598

HEALTH INSPECTORATE WALES

http://www.hiw.org.uk/
Healthcare Inspectorate Wales
Bevan House, Caerphilly Business Park
Van Road, Caerphilly CF83 3ED
029 2092 8850

CARE STANDARDS INSPECTORATE WALES

http://www.csiw.wales.gov.uk/index.asp
National Office
4/5 Charnwood Court
Heol Billingsley, Parc Nantgarw
Nantgarw CF15 7QZ
01443 848450

OTHER USEFUL WEBSITES

TRADING STANDARDS
http://www.tradingstandards.gov.uk/

SURGICAL AESTHETICS
www.surgicalaesthetics.com

WEST LONDON CLINIC
www.westlondonclinic.co.uk

THE CONSULTING ROOM
www.consultingroom.com

AMERICAN BOARD OF PLASTIC SURGERY
http://www.abplsurg.org/

AMERICAN SOCIETY OF AESTHETIC PLASTIC SURGEONS
http://www.surgery.org/

INTERNATIONAL SOCIETY OF AESTHETIC PLASTIC SURGERY
http://www.isaps.org/

INTERNATIONAL SOCIETY OF DERMATOLOGY
http://www.intsocdermatol.org/

BRITISH INSTITUTE AND ASSOCIATION OF ELECTROLYSIS
www.electrolysis.co.uk
0870 128 0477

A GUIDE TO CHOOSING A COSMETIC SURGEON

When you are considering cosmetic surgery, you should not underestimate the gravity of what you are investigating. Essentially, what you are thinking about is to alter, in some way, the reflection you see when you look in the mirror. For ever. It is therefore absolutely vital that you take your time to find the right cosmetic surgeon for you. This is the only face or body you have: surely you want to take every precaution possible so that you can be confident that you will get the best result that is achievable?

A WORD ABOUT COSMETIC SURGERY ON THE NHS The National Health Service is under huge financial restraints, and, as a result of this, cosmetic surgery procedures are largely unavailable through the NHS. However, some procedures can be justifiable in the NHS if there is a demonstrable need for it for psychological and physical reasons. Whether these will be considered or even carried out will vary from region to region, and will depend upon financial status and current policies. Some procedures, such as breast reduction, do sometimes fall within the scope of the NHS because they have a significant impact on the physical and psychological well-being of some individuals.

RESEARCH, RESEARCH, RESEARCH

The success of your cosmetic surgery depends in a large part on the skill of the person performing the operation. And all surgery carries risks – therefore, when you are looking for someone to perform your surgery privately, you need to find someone who is suitably qualified, is experienced and has a good professional reputation. You will also need to have faith in their ability to make a good aesthetic judgement on your behalf during surgery. The only way to get this confidence in your surgeon is to do your research.

Talk to your GP about the fact that you are thinking about having cosmetic surgery. They will be able to explain more and let you know if there might be provision for the operation on the NHS. They might also be able to refer you to a surgeon. Although the fact that they are recommended by your GP is obviously a good thing, you shouldn't be afraid to apply the quality controls listed in this chapter to this surgeon as you would to any other.

THE SPECIALIST SURGEON'S QUALIFICATIONS

I have put together the following checklist to help you find the best surgeon for your procedure. We'll start with ensuring that the practitioner is suitably qualified. The first thing you should do before you head for a consultation is to check that the person who will be performing your operation is registered as a physician (medical doctor) with the General Medical Council (GMC). You can do this by phoning them or by checking on their website – their details can be found on page 322.

DOCTORS

There are a number of levels of expertise that the practitioner offering you cosmetic surgery can have. In the UK, it is legal for a qualified physician (medical doctor) to carry out cosmetic surgery procedures. Nevertheless, I personally do not feel that you should leave the delicate task of your operation to someone who is only qualified as a physician. I would always suggest that you seek only the most qualified and expert surgeons in the procedure you are considering, so that you can be confident that you are in the very best hands available. It is my belief that your cosmetic surgery should only be carried out by qualified surgeons who are registered as specialists in Plastic Surgery, General Surgery, Maxillofacial or Ear, Nose and Throat with the General Medical Council.

IN THE KNOW You might also find it useful to consult newspapers, books and magazines, in particular the latest trade press journals devoted to cosmetic surgery, to see who is being asked for their opinion. However, you shouldn't use this method alone to find a surgeon, as it doesn't always follow that the most visible surgeons or practices are the experts in their field.

SPECIALIST SURGEONS

Surgeons who are specialists in the above areas are highly trained physicians who have undertaken many years of specialist training, gathered many hours of surgical experience and taken examinations in the subject. It stands to reason that these are the practitioners you should seek, as they hold some of the highest qualifications in the field and are likely to have the greatest amount of experience in surgical procedures. You should also check that the surgeon holds the correct 'privileges' to operate at an accredited hospital. Privileges are the regularly reviewed rights of a surgeon to operate at a hospital. Many high-quality private hospitals will provide you with a list of the surgeons who have operating privileges for that establishment.

THE SPECIALIST SURGEON'S EXPERIENCE

Now we'll look at how to find the most experienced surgeon. If your surgeon is suitably experienced, they will be only too happy to provide details relating to the number of times they have been in surgery. As a rough guide, in my twenty-two years of performing cosmetic surgery, I have performed more than ten thousand operations. Always ask to see a copy of your surgeon's CV, if you are not sure who you are dealing with. The more they have been in the operating theatre, the more likely they are to be familiar with the technique and possible complications, which puts them in a better position to expertly treat you. The experienced surgeon will also be able to detail how they keep abreast of the latest developments in the field through attendance at medical conferences relating to their specialities. Finally, they will be able to provide you with plenty of before-and-after photographs of previous work.

THE SPECIALIST SURGEON'S PROFESSIONAL REPUTATION

Once we know that they are well qualified and that they have experience, we should consider their professional reputation. Even if you have found a surgeon with a specialization in cosmetic surgery and who has plenty of surgical experience, there are still many different types of cosmetic surgical operations, each with their own developing technologies and changes in best practice.

Considering this, you might want to look for the individuals who are the leading experts in the operation you require. The way to do this is to research the names of the people who are writing books on the subject, are writing and presenting papers at medical conferences on the operations, and are members of the professional bodies such as the British Association of Aesthetic Plastic Surgeons (BAAPS) or, in the United States, the American Board of Plastic Surgery (ABPS). There are many such organizations listed on pages 323–5.

> TALKING TO PAST PATIENTS Once you have satisfied yourself that you have found the right person to perform your surgery, you may want to further supplement your research by talking to past patients and hearing their testimonials. For a first-hand account of what it is like to undergo surgery with the surgeon you are considering, ask to speak to one or two of their past patients. This can be a very useful and impartial way to find out what it's really like.

OTHER FACTORS

If you follow the above checklist, you should be able to find the practitioner you can have the most confidence in – the practitioner you can trust to be the best aesthetic judge during surgery. However, as you know, it is not only the surgeon's skill you need to have faith in, but also the team that surrounds them and the place where the operation will take happen.

THE SURGEON'S CLINIC

It is likely that once you have drawn up a shortlist of potential surgeons for your operation, the first thing you will do will be to call their clinic. You should start assessing the surgeon's practice the minute you get an answer. Be wary of the clinic that is too pushy, too abrupt or too patronizing. You could be speaking to the practice a lot after your surgery, particularly if you have any complications or suspect an infection, so if you get a response you don't like, move on to the next on the list.

You might also want to consider the location of the clinic, as it will be the focus of your aftercare. It should be reasonably close to home, or you should at least be able to stay nearby in case you need to be seen quickly in the post-operative period.

Remember, too, that a fast appointment to see the surgeon is not always just a sign of efficient service. In fact, it is more often the case that you have to wait for an appointment with an experienced and busy surgeon. If you book a consultation, use your common sense when you arrive. Make sure that the clinic is clean, and that the receptionists and nurses are professional and personable.

THE CONSULTATION

I would recommend that you have more than one consultation about your surgery. Expect to pay a fee for this. In fact, you should be wary of any practitioner who offers free consultations. Similarly, you should always make sure that you are seen by the person who will be performing your treatment; most surgeons will insist on this as a matter of course.

During the consultation, your practitioner will do all of the following:
- Ask you what you would like to change about your appearance
- Review the options available to you
- Discuss your medical history
- Discuss the potential risks and the potential benefits of the procedure
- Discuss the procedure – what will happen before, during and after surgery
- Examine you and assess your suitability

- Recommend the procedure(s) they consider to be right for you
- Show you before-and-after photographs of past patients

They may also do the following:
- With your permission, take photographs for before-and-after material, and conduct digital imaging so you can get an idea of what surgery might do (you'll get an idea of their aesthetic skills from this, too). Make sure you let your surgeon know if you are unhappy about anyone else seeing these photos.
- Take measurements and draw on you to show you where the incisions will be
- Ask you to have a blood test to screen for infectious diseases

A consultation is a two-way process, so you may wish to have prepared your own set of questions about the process; and you can always take notes. This way, you can be sure that you get all the answers you need at the meeting. You may also want to take along a friend for support during the consultation. Don't be afraid to ask the surgeon about their rates of revision surgery – i.e. the need for more than one trip to the operating theatre to achieve a good result – and what happens if you are not happy after the operation. You can also ask to see a copy of the results of any recent audits or inspections, which the clinic (and the surgeon) may have been through. Remember that the best will only be too happy to give you this information, so you shouldn't be worried about requesting it.

It is very important that you trust your instincts during a consultation. The best cosmetic surgeon will inspire confidence during a consultation, take time to answer all of your questions, understand and appreciate your concerns, and be pleasant and personable. Never tolerate a 'you leave it to me' attitude. Cosmetic surgery can be an emotional rollercoaster, and you shouldn't underestimate the importance of a good bedside manner.

THE HOSPITAL

You should also research the location where your practitioner is proposing to conduct the treatment. Ask for a list of surgeons who have operating privileges in their establishment – the reputations of the surgeons who use the hospital are often a good indication of the calibre of the hospital. Also ask about rates of MRSA or other infections at the hospital, and read up on how long the hospital has performed surgery, who it is funded by and how many patients have passed through its doors.

THE COST

When you ask about fees for your surgery, make sure that the clinic is absolutely clear about how much the entire procedure will cost.

Check to see if the fee that you have been quoted includes the following or whether it will be itemized or charged separately:

- Hospital
- Operating theatre and equipment
- Anaesthetist
- Nurse's fees
- Revision surgery
- Follow-up appointments
- Medication/dressings
- Administration charges

Cosmetic surgery is not an inexpensive business, but you should be very wary if the cost of the procedure is your greatest consideration. While it is reasonably safe to assume that the cheapest surgery is unlikely to be the best, neither is great expense necessarily a guarantee of quality. Packages of procedures will probably work out cheaper in the long run, but in general I would recommend that a small procedure with an excellent surgeon is always going to provide better value for money than a cheaper quote for a full face overhaul.

Private cosmetic surgery is now a multi-million pound business, which can make the field difficult to navigate, particularly if you are new to it and are willing to believe the hype. My advice is always to approach cosmetic surgery with realistic expectations and a practical attitude, having done plenty of research to find the best surgeon or nurses, hospital or clinic, for you. Your experience should then be one of a professional, efficient service with demonstrable improvements to both your appearance and psychological well-being.

OVERSEAS DOCTORS It is possible that your doctor or surgeon might have taken their medical examinations abroad and therefore not hold the qualifications listed above. However, if their qualifications and experience have been assessed as suitable and they are entitled to practise in this country, they will be registered with the General Medical Council. Furthermore, the GMC will always explain the nature of a physician's registration so that you can fully understand the nature of your practitioner's medical training.

ADVERTS FOR COSMETIC SURGERY Advertisements for cosmetic surgery are everywhere: on TV, in magazines and especially on the internet. Be aware that adverts are exactly that: they are selling cosmetic surgery services to you. I would always recommend that you retain a healthy dose of scepticism when considering these adverts. They may well be a good place to start when compiling a shortlist of potential clinics and surgeons, but always investigate them further before signing up for surgery. The best will stand up to scrutiny, and those that don't are the ones that are better left behind.

A GUIDE TO MEDICAL QUALIFICATIONS

The following guide should give you an understanding of what you might come across when you are investigating the qualifications of your practitioner.

DOCTORS

There are five years of medical training and medical exams to pass before a student can provisionally register with the General Medical Council as a physician (medical doctor). Following provisional registration, a doctor spends a year in a hospital as a pre-registration house officer, after which time they will register as a fully qualified physician with the GMC. This level of expertise is signified by the medical qualifications MBBS, BM BCh or MBChB, which means Bachelor of Medicine and Bachelor of Surgery.

SURGEONS

Surgeons are qualified medical doctors who choose to specialize in surgery. After they fully qualify as a doctor with the GMC, these doctors spend a further five or more years studying surgery. Once they have completed this study and successfully passed the surgical exams, they qualify as a surgeon. This level of expertise is indicated by the letters: FRCS – Fellow of the Royal College of Surgeons England, FRCS (Ed) – Fellow of the Royal College of Surgeons Edinburgh, FRCS (Glas) – Fellow of the Royal College of Surgeons Glasgow, FRCSI – Fellow of the Royal College of Surgeons Ireland.

In addition to this, surgeons will spend around another five years gaining surgical experience to train as specialists (equivalent to Consultant level in the NHS) in a particular type of surgery. For example, a further speciality in Plastic Surgery would be signified by the letters FRCSPlast. There are a number of these specialities: other examples are FRCS (GenSurg), which means General Surgery, and FRCS (OFMS), which means Oral and Maxillofacial Surgery. Currently no speciality of this sort exists for cosmetic surgery, so expertise in this field is largely defined by a combination of qualifications, experience, professional reputation and referrals.

ANAESTHETISTS

An anaesthetist is a qualified physician who has taken seven further years specialist training and passed exams in anaesthesia. If they do this, they will have FRCA after their name.

DERMATOLOGISTS

A dermatologist is a qualified physician who has specialized in diagnosing and treating diseases of the skin, hair and nails. They are usually signified by the following qualification: FRCP or MRCP (Fellow/Member of the Royal College of Physicians).

NURSES

To qualify as a nurse in the UK, you need to undertake three years of training which will include a specialism in either adult, children's, mental health or learning disability nursing. The following letters after a nurse's name indicate that they are a qualified nurse: RN (Registered Nurse), RGN (Registered General Nurse) or BA (Hons)/ BSc/Diploma in Nursing. There is a qualification register for nurses held by the Nursing and Midwifery Council. Following qualification, nurses can undertake any of a number of further specializations, such as attending courses in non-surgical cosmetic treatments. Always check the training your nurse specifies with the certifying body listed so you can be confident that your nurse is suitably trained. Suitably qualified and experienced practitioners will be only too happy to provide evidence.

OTHER COURSES

Many manufacturers of specific machines or products offer training courses to practitioners to train and equip them to use the machine or product in accordance with the manufacturer's specifications. Although these courses often give the practitioner a course certificate, this is not something that is regulated or checked. Before embarking on any treatment, you still need to get specific details about what training course your practitioner attended, what was covered during the course and what subsequent experience they have had with the machine or product since the training.

WHAT TO DO IF THE RESULTS OF YOUR SURGERY ARE NOT WHAT YOU EXPECT

As you know by now, there are no guarantees with cosmetic surgery. If you have been realistic about what can be achieved, you will probably be pleased with the results you get. There will always be times when the results are unexpected, but a bad result owing to complications or unrealistic expectations is an entirely different thing from a bad result through mistreatment or lack of informed consent. Although complications are very rare, they do happen. Some are just a bit unsightly and temporary, but others can be painful and permanent. Most complications will be an unfortunate side effect that you will have been made aware could happen, since it is impossible for the surgeon to completely predict how your body will react to surgery before it happens. In these cases, complications really are down to bad luck. You need to keep this in the front of your mind before you head for the operating theatre: although the surgeon will try their best to prevent complications from occurring, it is not always possible.

THE FIRST STEP: GO BACK TO YOUR SURGEON

If you don't like a shirt you have bought, you take it back to the shop. You don't contact the Financial Ombudsman and immediately start proceedings. You should apply the same logic with your surgeon. Most surgeons would want to talk to a patient who is unhappy with the result of their surgery. Many, but not all, will offer a revision operation free of charge (you'll still have to pay for the extras such as the hospital and anaesthetist, though) if they agree that the results are not ideal. This way, in many cases, complaints are resolved. Be aware, however, that most surgeons will ask you to wait until the scars have completely settled (which could take up to a year) before they consider another operation.

Some surgeons may not want to do a revision operation themselves, but may offer the services of a colleague. This can also be good if you have lost faith in the ability of your original surgeon, and it is for this reason that some surgeons consider this a preferable route. Make sure it is absolutely clear from the outset who will bear the cost of this extra operation.

THE NEXT STEP: MAKE A COMPLAINT

If you are unhappy with how the surgeon, nurse, hospital or clinic has dealt with your complaint, there are a number of organizations you can contact to complain about the treatment you have received. To complain about a surgeon or doctor, contact the General Medical Council. To complain about a nurse, contact the Nursing and Midwifery Council. To complain about a clinic or hospital, contact the Healthcare Commission; if an establishment fails to meet their standards, they can take action against them. You can also complain to Trading Standards. You can report any adverse effects of medicines or machines to the Medicines and Healthcare products Regulatory Agency (MHRA). There is also a body called the Independent Sector Complaints Adjudication Service to which you can complain if your practitioner is a member. You will find the numbers for these organizations on pages 322–5.

THE LAST RESORT: CONSIDER LEGAL ACTION

If you believe you didn't consent to the operation performed or you suspect that the surgeon was negligent, legal action is a possibility. However, it can be a lengthy and prohibitively expensive business, so you need to be absolutely sure that you have a good case before you begin any action. You are much more likely to have just cause if you weren't made aware that the complication you have suffered was a potential risk of surgery, or if the surgeon performed an operation on you without your informed consent. Three years is the normal window of time in which you can bring a complaint.

A charity that can help you contact a solicitor who specializes in medical cases is Action for Victims of Medical Accidents (see page 324). A solicitor will advise you further about the charges you can bring and whether you have a legitimate cause for complaint. If your case does go to court, it is likely that the advice you were given will be scrutinized and the opinion of an independent surgeon will be sought.

However, if you carefully consider your options, do your research to find a great surgeon and team, are fit and healthy and have realistic expectations, you should get a good result from your surgery and thus have no reason at all to complain. Remember that, for the vast majority, their cosmetic surgery operations go very smoothly indeed.

GOING ABROAD FOR COSMETIC SURGERY

It is possible to go abroad for your cosmetic surgery. In fact, it can be considerably cheaper if you go to another country, and some of the very best surgeons can be accessed by trying further afield.

Although it might be tempting to have surgery done cheaply at some faraway beautiful place, there are disadvantages with going abroad for your surgery.

Most importantly, you should be aware that not all countries have the same standards of hygiene, and regulation differs from country to country. What is considered clean in one hospital is not always acceptable elsewhere. You need to apply the same high standards you would use in assessing a British establishment.

Having done this, you also need to consider the following:
- How are surgeons in the country trained? How does the qualification compare with the UK?
- Who regulates the surgeon, hospital and nursing staff in that country?
- Does the surgeon or nurse fully understand my concerns and wishes, bearing in mind that sometimes surgeons abroad might not speak English?

- How do the standards of this surgeon or nurse, hospital or clinic, compare with those of the UK?
- Does this surgeon or nurse, hospital or clinic, have appropriate insurance in case something goes wrong? Does it cover people who are not citizens of that country?
- What happens if there are complications when I get home? Who can I go to? Will my GP be prepared to help?
- Can I afford the cost of an unexpected return visit that might be needed?

Factor in the added complication of travel and somewhat uncontrollable variables that are involved in going abroad for your cosmetic surgery and it might well affect your final decision.

GLOSSARY

ABDOMINOPLASTY
Surgical procedure to remove excess skin and tissue from the stomach area.

ABLATION
Removing the outer layers of the skin through vaporizing them.

ACNE
Inflammatory condition characterized by eruption of the skin.

ALLOGRAFT
Same species graft of tissue or skin.

ALPHA HYDROXY ACIDS (AHAS)
Fruit acids that brighten the complexion by helping to remove the outermost layer of the skin and promoting cell renewal.

ANAESTHETIC
Medication to cause loss of sensation or consciousness

ANTIHISTAMINE
Medication used to reduce skin itching.

AREOLA
The pigmented area around the nipple.

AUTOLOGOUS
Originating from the same individual into which it has been transferred.

BIOSKINJETTING
Cosmetic procedure in which cells in the epidermis and dermis are agitated to stimulate the production of collagen.

BLEPHAROPLASTY
An operation to remove excess tissue and fat from around the eyelids.

BODY DYSMORPHIC DISORDER
Psychological disorder where patients are inappropriately concerned with their appearance. People with BDD are not suitable for cosmetic surgery or procedures, in most cases.

BOTOX
Brand name for botulinum toxin, a muscle-relaxing medication.

BOVINE
Derived from cows.

BRACHIAPLASTY
Surgical operation to remove excess skin from the upper arms.

BROW LIFT
Surgery to move the brow to a higher position.

BUCCAL FAT
Fat from the inside of the lower cheek.

CADAVER
Dead person.

CANNULA
Long, thin tubular device used to extract fat during liposuction.

CAPILLARIES
Tiny arteries that convey nutrients around the body.

CAPSULAR CONTRACTURE
A complication that can occur with implants, where scar tissue forms so tightly around the implant that it contracts into a hard lump.

CARBON DIOXIDE LASER
A laser that removes the outermost layers of the skin. It can also be used as a cutting tool in surgery.

CELLULITE
Deposits of fat that cause a dimpled appearance in the skin.

CHEMICAL PEEL
Skin resurfacing achieved through the application of acid or other irritants on the face.

CLOSTRIDIUM BOTULINUM
The bacteria that is used to create botulinum toxin injections.

COLLAGEN
Component of skin that gives it structure and tone. The body produces less as we age.

CONTRAINDICATION
Any existing illness, allergy or condition

that significantly affects the risks posed by a procedure, thus making it inadvisable to proceed.

CROTON OIL
Oil extracted from the croton plant used as an agent in deep peeling.

CROW'S FEET
Wrinkles around the eyes.

D

DERMABRASION
A form of skin resurfacing that uses a scraping action to remove the outer layers of the skin.

DERMAL FILLER
Injectables used to plump out specific wrinkles in the face.

DERMAPLANING
Skin resurfacing using the scraping action of a surgical blade.

DERMATOLOGY
Relating to the study of skin.

DERMIS
The layer of skin underneath the epidermis where collagen and elastin are present.

DRY EYE
A condition of the eyelid caused by low tear production, characterized by dryness, irritation and swelling of the eyes.

DVT
Deep vein thrombosis. A serious condition caused by the presence of a blood clot in the leg.

DYNAMIC RHYTID
Wrinkles associated with movements made by the face.

E

ELASTIN
Connective tissue that exists alongside collagen to support the structure of the skin.

ELECTROLYSIS
A process of removing hair by passing an electric current into the hair follicle to heat it and cause damage that stops the

follicle from producing any more hair.

ENDOSCOPE
A small, rigid, tubular instrument which can be inserted in the body through a tiny incision and which lights up an area to show on a TV monitor while the surgeon performs the operation.

EPIDERMIS
The outermost layer of the skin.

ERBIUM:YAG LASER SKIN RESURFACING
A type of laser resurfacing where the outermost layers of the skin are removed.

ERYTHEMA
Skin redness caused by an increase in blood supply to the skin.

EXCISION
Surgical cutting to remove.

EXFOLIANT
A granular material that removes dead skin cells when applied to the face.

EXTRINSIC AGEING
Ageing of the skin caused by the environment, such as the sun.

EXTRUSION
Exposure of an implant caused by the erosion of skin and tissue.

F

FACELIFT
Surgical operation to reposition and remove excess facial skin that contributes to ageing.

FAT TRANSFER
Surgical procedure whereby fat is taken from one part of the body and injected into another as a filler.

FIBROBLAST
Cells that form collagen fibres in the skin.

FRACTIONAL LASER RESURFACING
A new type of laser resurfacing that works on a fraction of the deeper layers of the skin at a time.

G

GENIOPLASTY
Surgical operation to alter the contour of

the chin bone.

GLABELLAR
Between the eyebrows.

GLYCOLIC ACID
A fruit acid used in superficial peels.

GRAFT
Tissue that is removed from one part of the body, transferred and attached to another.

GRANULOMA
A lump of firm tissue that forms as a reaction to the presence of a foreign body.

GYNECOMASTIA
The presence of excess breast tissue in males.

H

HAEMATOMA
Localized accumulation of clotted blood. One of the more common complications of surgery.

HYPERPIGMENTATION
Darkening of skin caused by excess pigment.

HYPOPIGMENTATION
Lightening of skin caused by lack of pigment.

I

INCISION
Cut in the skin and tissue made to perform surgery.

INFECTION
Localized collection of bacteria. One of the more common complications of surgery.

INTRINSIC AGEING
Ageing that occurs from within the body as a natural consequence of getting older and inheritance.

IPL
Intense pulsed light treatment. A form of light energy used for rejuvenating skin and removing hair.

J

JOWLS
The collection of skin around the jawline that occurs as a consequence of the skin on the face gradually slipping with age.

K

KELOID
Fibrous scar tissue that doesn't stop growing.

L

LABIAPLASTY
Surgical procedure to alter the shape of the labia (folds of the vulva).

LASER
Acronym for Light Amplification by the Stimulated Emission of Radiation. An intense energy beam of light that can be easily and directly controlled.

LASER SKIN RESURFACING
Laser removal of superficial skin for treatment of skin conditions.

LIGNOCAINE
A common local anaesthetic.

LIPOSUCTION
The removal of fat from the body using a small hollow instrument called a cannula.

M

MALARPLASTY
Surgical procedure to place an implant into the cheek to change the volume and shape.

MAMMAPLASTY
Surgical change of breast volume and shape.

MANDIBLE
Referring to the lower jaw.

MARIONETTE LINES
The vertical wrinkles that form from the corners of the mouth to the jowls.

MASK LIFT
Surgery to lift all of the facial structures at a depth just above the bone.

MASTOPEXY
Surgical operation to lift the breast.

MAXILLARY
Referring to the upper jaw.
MELANIN
The pigment that protects skin from UV damage.
MELASMA
Localized melanin overproduction, probably hormone-related.
MENTOPLASTY
Surgical procedure to alter the chin.
MESOTHERAPY
An alternative form of therapy where a vitamin mixture is injected into the skin to rejuvenate.
MICRO-CURRENT TREATMENT
A skin-rejuvenating procedure where tiny electric currents are passed through the skin. It is thought that this will stimulate collagen production.
MICRODERMABRASION
The process of firing tiny crystals at the skin to remove the outermost layers of the skin.
MICROPIGMENTATION
Also called dermagraphics. Semi-permanent pigment is inserted into the lower levels of the skin to create the appearance of make-up or to cover blemishes or scars.
MICROSCLEROTHERAPY
As sclerotherapy, but the specific technique used to treat facial thread veins.
MICRO-THERMOCOAGULATION TREATMENT
A procedure in which heat is applied to the dermis to stimulate the production of collagen in the skin.
MILIA
Tiny cysts that may appear on the skin after laser resurfacing or close to scars.
N
NASAO- LABIAL FOLD
The fold that extends from the nose to the mouth.
NECROSIS
Cell death due to lack of blood supply.

O
OEDEMA
Post-operative swelling or fluid retention.
OTOPLASTY
Also called pinnaplasty. Surgical procedure to pin back ears.
P
PARAFFIN
Waxy solid substance used to make candles, a one-time dermal filler.
PHALLOPLASTY
Surgical procedures to alter the size of the penis.
PHENOL
Deep-peel agent.
PHLEBITIS
Vein inflammation.
PHOTODAMAGE
Damage of the skin that can be attributed to the effects of the sun.
PHOTOREJUVENATION
The use of light to rejuvenate the face.
PLASMA SKIN RESURFACING
The use of plasma to rejuvenate the face.
POST-OPERATIVE
After surgery.
PTOSIS
Clinical word for drooping.
R
RADIOFREQUENCY
The use of radiofrequency waves to rejuvenate the face.
RESORCINOL
A peeling agent.
RHINOPLASTY
Surgical procedure to alter the contour and size of the nose.
RHYTIDECTOMY
Clinical term for a facelift.
RHYTIDS
Clinical name for wrinkles.
ROSACEA
Skin complaint that is characterized by redness, spots and enlarged blood vessels.

S

SCAR
A permanent mark on the skin as a result of trauma to the skin.

SCLERAL SHOW
A potential complication of eyelid surgery where the white part of the eyeball is left permanently exposed.

SCLEROTHERAPY
The process of injecting thread veins with a chemical that causes them to collapse and therefore disappear.

SEBACEOUS GLANDS
Clinical term for sweat glands.

SEROMA
Localized collection of clear fluid that may occur during and after surgery.

SILICONE
A synthetic substance used in breast and body implants and as a filler.

SMAS
Acronym for Superficial Musculo Aponeurotic System. A tissue layer that covers the deeper structures of the cheek.

SPF
Sun Protection Factor.

SPIDER VEIN
A spider-like group of tiny veins that are visible on the surface of the skin.

STATIC RHYTID
Wrinkle associated with external factors, such as the sun.

SUBCUTANEOUS
Under the skin.

SUBMENTAL
The area below the chin.

SUBPERIOSTEAL
The term for a procedure that goes deep into the layers of tissue under the skin; under the lining of the bone.

SUTURE
Stitches: fibres used to sew together parts of the body.

T

TELANGIECTASIA
Clinical term for thread veins.

THIGHPLASTY
Surgical procedure to remove excess skin and tissue from the thighs.

THREAD LIFT
Also called suture facelift and contour lift. A procedure where small threads are placed into the subcutaneous tissue of the face and tension is placed upon the threads to produce a lift.

THREAD VEIN
Tiny veins that are visible on the surface of the skin.

TUMESCENT
Large volume of anaethestic and saline (salt water) solution is injected to swell and desensitize the operating area.

U

ULTRASOUND
A soundwave vibration of more than 16,000 cycles a second; inaudible sound.

UMBILICOPLASTY
Surgical procedure to alter the contours of the belly button

V

VAGINOPLASTY
Surgical procedures to alter the vagina.

VARICOSE VEINS
Rope-like swollen veins that appear in the legs as a result of poor circulation.

VASCULAR
Referring to the channel used for the conveyance of bodily fluid; i.e. blood vessels.

VERMILION BORDER
The outer pinkish border of the lips.

VITILIGO
Loss of skin pigment due to autoimmune causes.

W

WRINKLE
A crease in the skin.

ACKNOWLEDGEMENTS

To my wife Sue and girls Nicola and Sophie, for your constant patience and unending support over the past few months, particularly during our holiday in Spain!

To Felix, for your humour and encouragement every day.

To Colette Foster, for the opportunity: I hope you like the result! Also for your objectivity, efficiency and continuous support throughout the months of writing.

To Sarah Emsley at Transworld, for your fantastic guidance, and laughing at all the right times and in all the right places!

To Alison Wormleighton, for being so thorough.

To Rachel Barke at RDF, for all your help and professionalism.

To all at Maverick, in particular Alex Fraser and Jim Sayer: and, of course, the production team of *10 Years Younger*, past and present. Without you there would be no book to write!

And finally, thank you to all the contributors to *10 Years Younger*, for helping us to demystify cosmetic surgery for the millions who watch the series on television.

INDEX